Updates in Cardiac MRI

Editor

KAREN G. ORDOVAS

MAGNETIC RESONANCE IMAGING CLINICS OF NORTH AMERICA

www.mri.theclinics.com

Consulting Editors
SURESH K. MUKHERJI
LYNNE S. STEINBACH

February 2015 • Volume 23 • Number 1

ELSEVIER

1600 John F. Kennedy Boulevard • Suite 1800 • Philadelphia, Pennsylvania, 19103-2899

http://www.mri.theclinics.com

MRI CLINICS OF NORTH AMERICA Volume 23, Number 1
February 2015 ISSN 1064-9689, ISBN 13: 978-0-323-35444-8

Editor: John Vassallo (j.vassallo@elsevier.com)
Developmental Editor: Barbara Cohen-Kligerman

Magnetic Resonance Imaging Clinics of North America (ISSN 1064-9689) is published quarterly by Elsevier Inc., 360 Park Avenue South, New York, NY 10010-1710. Months of issue are February, May, August, and November. Business and Editorial Offices: 1600 John F. Kennedy Blvd., Ste. 1800, Philadelphia, PA 19103-2899. Customer Service Office: 3251 Riverport Lane, Maryland Heights, MO 63043. Periodicals postage paid at New York, NY and additional mailing offices. Subscription prices are $375.00 per year (domestic individuals), $581.00 per year (domestic institutions), $190.00 per year (domestic students/residents), $420.00 per year (Canadian individuals), $755.00 per year (Canadian institutions), $545.00 per year (international individuals), $755.00 per year (international institutions), and $275.00 per year (international and Canadian students/residents). International air speed delivery is included in all *Clinics* subscription prices. All prices are subject to change without notice. **POSTMASTER:** Send address changes to *Magnetic Resonance Imaging Clinics*, Elsevier Health Sciences Division, Subscription Customer Service, 3251 Riverport Lane, Maryland Heights, MO 63043. Customer Service (orders, claims, online, change of address): Elsevier Health Sciences Division, Subscription Customer Service, 3251 Riverport Lane, Maryland Heights, MO 63043. Tel:1-800-654-2452 (U.S. and Canada); 314-447-8871 (outside U.S. and Canada). Fax: 314-447-8029. E-mail: journalscustomerservice-usa@elsevier.com (for print support); journalsonlinesupport-usa@elsevier.com (for online support).

Reprints. For copies of 100 or more of articles in this publication, please contact the Commercial Reprints Department, Elsevier Inc., 360 Park Avenue South, New York, NY 10010-1710. Tel.: 212-633-3874; Fax: 212-633-3820; E-mail: reprints@elsevier.com.

Magnetic Resonance Imaging Clinics of North America is covered in the *RSNA Index of Imaging Literature, MEDLINE/PubMed (Index Medicus),* and *EMBASE/Excerpta Medica.*

Contributors

CONSULTING EDITORS

SURESH K. MUKHERJI, MD, MBA, FACR
Professor and Chairman; W.F. Patenge
Endowed Chair, Department of Radiology,
Michigan State University, East Lansing,
Michigan

LYNNE S. STEINBACH, MD, FACR
Professor of Clinical Radiology and
Orthopaedic Surgery, Department of
Radiology and Biomedical Imaging, University
of California San Francisco, San Francisco,
California

EDITOR

KAREN G. ORDOVAS, MD, MAS
Associate Professor in Residence, Department
of Radiology and Biomedical Imaging;
Director of Cardiac Imaging, University of
California San Francisco, San Francisco,
California

AUTHORS

PRACHI P. AGARWAL, MBBS, MS
Division of Cardiothoracic Radiology,
Department of Radiology, University of
Michigan, Ann Arbor, Michigan

SPENCER C. BEHR, MD
Assistant Professor of Clinical Radiology,
Department of Radiology and Biomedical
Imaging, University of California San Francisco,
San Francisco, California

MAURICE B. BIZINO, MD
Department of Radiology, Leiden University
Medical Center, Leiden, The Netherlands

NICHOLAS S. BURRIS, MD
Department of Radiology and Biomedical
Imaging, University of California San Francisco,
San Francisco, California

DANIELLE CHAN, MD
Department of Radiology, Indiana University,
Indianapolis, Indiana

PIERLUIGI CIET, MD
Fellow, Department of Radiology, Beth Israel
Deaconess Medical Center, Boston,
Massachusetts; Department of Radiology,
Erasmus Medical Center; Department of
Pediatrics, Respiratory Medicine and Allergy,
Erasmus Medical Center-Sophia Children's
Hospital, Rotterdam, The Netherlands

PAUL DE HEER, MSc
C.J. Gorter Center for High Field MRI,
Department of Radiology, Leiden University
Medical Center, Leiden, The Netherlands

ALBERT DE ROOS, MD, PhD
Department of Radiology, Leiden University
Medical Center, Leiden, The Netherlands

ADAM L. DORFMAN, MD
Division of Pediatric Cardiology, Department of
Pediatrics and Communicable Diseases;
Division of Pediatric Radiology, Department of
Radiology, University of Michigan, Ann Arbor,
Michigan

JULIANO LARA FERNANDES, MD, MBA, PhD
Cardiovascular Imaging Center, Jose Michel
Kalaf Research Institute, Campinas, São Paulo,
Brazil

ROBERT GROVES, MD
Department of Radiology, Virginia
Commonwealth University, Richmond, Virginia

HENRIK HARALDSSON, PhD
Department of Radiology and Biomedical
Imaging, University of California San Francisco,
San Francisco, California

CHARLES B. HIGGINS, MD
Department of Radiology, Cardiac and
Pulmonary Imaging, University of California
San Francisco, San Francisco, California

MICHAEL D. HOPE, MD
Department of Radiology and Biomedical
Imaging, University of California San Francisco,
San Francisco, California

MASAKI ISHIDA, MD
Department of Radiology, Mie University
Hospital, Tsu, Mie, Japan

KIMBERLY KALLIANOS, MD
Resident Physician, Department of Radiology
and Biomedical Imaging, University of
California San Francisco, San Francisco,
California

NAZIMA N. KATHIRIA, DO
Department of Radiology, Cardiac and
Pulmonary Imaging, University of California
San Francisco, San Francisco, California

SUMA H. KONETY, MD, MS
Division of Cardiology, University of Minnesota
Medical Center, Minneapolis, Minnesota

HILDEBRANDUS J. LAMB, MD, PhD
Department of Radiology, Leiden University
Medical Center, Leiden, The Netherlands

DIANA E. LITMANOVICH, MD
Assistant Professor, Harvard Medical School;
Department of Radiology, Beth Israel
Deaconess Medical Center, Boston,
Massachusetts

JING LIU, PhD
Department of Radiology and Biomedical
Imaging, University of California San Francisco,
San Francisco, California

MARIA CLARA N. LORCA, MD
Department of Radiology and Biomedical
Imaging, University of California San Francisco,
San Francisco, California

JIMMY C. LU, MD
Division of Pediatric Cardiology, Department of
Pediatrics and Communicable Diseases;
Division of Pediatric Radiology, Department of
Radiology, University of Michigan, Ann Arbor,
Michigan

MARYAM GHADIMI MAHANI, MD
Divisions of Pediatric Radiology and
Cardiothoracic Radiology, Department of
Radiology, University of Michigan, Ann Arbor,
Michigan

CAROLINA MASRI, MD
Division of Cardiology, University of
Washington Medical Center, Seattle,
Washington

GUSTAVO L. MORAES, MD
Assistant Professor of Clinical Radiology,
Department of Radiology, Hospital Mae de
Deus, Porto Alegre, Rio Grande do Sul,
Brazil

DAVID M. NAEGER, MD
Assistant Professor of Clinical Radiology,
Department of Radiology and Biomedical
Imaging, University of California San Francisco,
San Francisco, California

KAREN G. ORDOVAS, MD, MAS
Associate Professor in Residence, Department
of Radiology and Biomedical Imaging;
Director of Cardiac Imaging, University of
California San Francisco, San Francisco,
California

CARLOS EDUARDO ROCHITTE, MD, PhD
CMR and CCT Section, Cardiology
Department, Heart Institute (InCor), University
of Sao Paulo Medical School, São Paulo,
Sao Paulo, Brazil

HAJIME SAKUMA, MD
Department of Radiology, Mie University
Hospital, Tsu, Mie, Japan

MICHAEL L. SALA, MD
Department of Radiology, Leiden University
Medical Center, Leiden, The Netherlands

DAVID SALONER, PhD
Department of Radiology and Biomedical Imaging, University of California San Francisco; Department of Veterans Affairs Medical Center, San Francisco, California

JAN W.A. SMIT, MD, PhD
Division of Endocrinology, Department of Medicine, Radboud University Medical Centre, Nijmegen, The Netherlands

BRANDON M. SMITH, MD
Division of Pediatric Cardiology, Department of Pediatrics and Communicable Diseases, University of Michigan, Ann Arbor, Michigan

ASHENAFI M. TAMENE, MD
Division of Cardiology, University of Minnesota Medical Center, Minneapolis, Minnesota

SHAWN D. TEAGUE, MD
Department of Radiology, Indiana University, Indianapolis, Indiana

PIETERNEL VAN DER TOL, MSc
Department of Radiology, Leiden University Medical Center, Leiden, The Netherlands

ANDREW G. WEBB, PhD
C.J. Gorter Center for High Field MRI, Department of Radiology, Leiden University Medical Center, Leiden, The Netherlands

MARIANNA ZAGUROVSKAYA, MD
Department of Radiology, Virginia Commonwealth University, Richmond, Virginia

STEFAN L. ZIMMERMAN, MD
Assistant Professor, The Russell H. Morgan Department of Radiology and Radiological Sciences, Johns Hopkins University School of Medicine, Baltimore, Maryland

Contents

The quality of the medical imaging is a key component for accurate disease diagnosis. Optimizing image quality while maintaining scan time efficiency and patient comfort is important for routine clinical MRIs. In this article, we review both practical and advanced techniques for achieving high image quality, especially focusing on optimizing the trade-offs between the image quality (such as signal-to-noise and spatial resolution) and acquisition time. We provide practical examples for optimizing the image quality and scan time.

Magnetic resonance assessment of regional myocardial function is a novel potentially important tool for early identification of cardiac pathology. Many cardiac magnetic resonance techniques have been developed for detection and quantification of regional strain abnormalities including steady-state free-precession CINE, tagging, displacement encoding with stimulated echoes, strain encoding imaging, and feature tracking. Potential clinical applications of magnetic resonance strain imaging include early detection of systolic dysfunction in heart failure patients with both ischemic and nonischemic etiologies.

Aortic disease is routinely monitored with anatomic imaging, but until the recent advent of 3-directional phase contrast MRI (4D) flow, blood flow abnormalities have gone undetected. 4D flow measures aortic hemodynamic markers quickly. Qualitative flow visualization has spurred the investigation of new quantitative markers. Flow displacement and wall shear stress can quantify the effects of valve-related aortic flow abnormalities. Markers of turbulent and viscous energy loss approximate the increased energetic burden on the ventricle in disease states. This article discusses magnetic resonance flow imaging and highlights new flow-related markers in the context of aortic valve disease, valve-related aortic disease, and aortic wall disease.

T1 mapping, one form of tissue characterization performed with a parametric approach, has been gaining rapid popularity, as different sequences have been developed to integrate image acquisition into a clinical routine. This technique allows fast progression from the basics of sequence development to its application in normal individuals and distinct diseases, sometimes overriding the more gradual steps taken with other cardiovascular magnetic resonance advances. In this review, the state-of-the-art in T1 mapping is examined, focusing on its techniques, sequences, comparison of native versus extracellular volume fraction measurements, and the current and future clinical applications of the method.

Many novel cardiac MR sequences can be used for assessment of adult patients with congenital heart disease. Although most of these techniques are still primarily used in the research arena, there are many potential applications in clinical practice. Advanced cardiac MR assessment of myocardial tissue characterization, flow hemodynamics, and myocardial strain are promising tools for diagnostic and prognostic assessment late after repair of congenital heart diseases.

The metabolic syndrome (MetS) is characterized by ectopic lipid accumulation. Magnetic resonance (MR) imaging and spectroscopy can quantify ectopic lipid accumulation. Consequences of MetS can be evaluated with MR on a whole-body level. In the liver, several techniques are used to quantify hepatic steatosis and differentiate stages of nonalcoholic fatty liver disease. Cardiac MR can quantify myocardial steatosis and associated complications. In the brain, magnetization transfer imaging and diffusion tensor imaging can detect microstructural brain damage. Various other organs can be assessed with MR. MR is a powerful tool to unravel whole-body MetS pathophysiology, monitor therapeutic efficacy, and establish prognosis.

Because of its lack of ionizing radiation, MR imaging is increasingly used for patients with cardiovascular disease, including young women. However, the risks related to the MR environment need to be acknowledged and prevented. For women, there are unique gender-related safety issues that are important to address in cardiovascular MR examinations. This article familiarizes radiologists with MR safety issues and current, evidence-based recommendations for specific situations such as pregnancy or lactation and imaging of women who have pelvic gynecologic devices such as intrauterine devices. Practical algorithms to minimize risk and increase MR safety for these women are suggested.

Arrhythmogenic right ventricular cardiomyopathy/dysplasia (ARVC/D) is a rare inherited cardiomyopathy characterized by fibrofatty replacement of the right ventricular myocardium and risk of sudden death from ventricular tachyarrhythmias. Cardiac magnetic resonance (MR) imaging plays an important role in the diagnostic evaluation of patients and family members suspected of having ARVC/D. This article discusses the epidemiology and pathophysiology of ARVC/D, reviews typical MR imaging findings and diagnostic criteria, and summarizes potential pitfalls in the MR imaging evaluation of patients suspected of having ARVC/D.

Abnormal thickening or rigidity of the pericardium may compromise normal cardiac function. This condition is known as pericardial constriction, or constrictive pericarditis. Several imaging modalities are used to evaluate the pericardium, including MR, computed tomography, and echocardiography, which can all play a complementary role aiding diagnosis. This article focuses on MR imaging and its role in the detection and evaluation of pericardial constriction. MR imaging has many advantages compared with other modalities including precise delineation of the pericardial thickness, evaluation of ventricular function, detection of wall motion abnormalities, and provision of information about common (and potentially harmful) sequelae of pericardial constriction.

The role of cardiac magnetic resonance (MR) imaging as a prognostic tool in patients with ischemic heart disease is well established. However, an increasing body of data now demonstrates that cardiac MR imaging can provide prognostic information in a variety of nonischemic and diffuse myocardial diseases including myocarditis, dilated and hypertrophic cardiomyopathies, sarcoidosis, amyloidosis, and arrhythmogenic right ventricular cardiomyopathy. Cardiac MR imaging can also supply incremental information above established prognostic indicators, providing an additional tool for use in the prediction of disease progression, response to treatment, and risk stratification.

PET and magnetic resonance (MR) imaging have each become essential tools in the workup and management of cardiac patients. Combined PET/MR systems have recently been developed, allowing for single-session imaging using both modalities. This new technology holds great promise for cardiac applications given the different, yet complementary, information each modality provides. Research in this area is still nascent, although early studies have been promising.

Patients with cancer are subject to short-term and long-term adverse cardiovascular outcomes from cancer therapies. It is important to identify patients at risk for cardiotoxicity so that appropriate therapy can be instituted early. Cardiovascular magnetic resonance (MR) imaging is emerging as a promising imaging modality with unique applications beyond standard left-ventricular systolic function assessment. It can provide comprehensive evaluation of most cardiac structures in one setting. This article provides an overview of cardiac MR imaging in cardio-oncology.

Magnetic resonance (MR) imaging of the coronary arteries has been challenging, owing to the small size of the vessels and the complex motion caused by cardiac contraction and respiration. Free-breathing, whole-heart coronary MR angiography has emerged as a method that can provide visualization of the entire coronary arterial tree within a single 3-dimensional acquisition. Although coronary MR angiography is noninvasive and without radiation exposure, acquisition of high-quality coronary images is operator dependent and is generally more difficult than computed tomographic angiography. This article explains how to optimize acquisition of coronary MR angiography for reliable assessment of coronary artery disease.

Vascular rings and pulmonary artery slings are rare congenital anomalies that often present with symptoms of tracheal and esophageal compression. These can involve the aortic arch branches and pulmonary arteries, respectively. This review illustrates the current role of MR imaging, highlights its advantages, and provides insight into the diagnosis of these anomalies by describing the embryology and characteristic imaging features of these lesions.

MAGNETIC RESONANCE IMAGING CLINICS OF NORTH AMERICA

RELATED INTEREST

Radiologic Clinics of North America, January 2014 (Vol. 52, No. 1)
Thoracic Imaging
Jane P. Ko, *Editor*

PROGRAM OBJECTIVE

The goal of *Magnetic Resonance Imaging Clinics of North America* is to keep practicing physicians up to date with current clinical practice by providing timely articles reviewing the state of the art in patient care.

TARGET AUDIENCE

All practicing physicians and healthcare professionals who provide patient care utilizing findings from Magnetic Resonance Imaging.

LEARNING OBJECTIVES

Upon completion of this activity, participants will be able to:
1. Discuss applications of PET-MRI for patients with cardiovascular disease.
2. Review cardiac MRI applications for cancer patients.
3. Describe MR safety issues pertaining to women.

ACCREDITATION

The Elsevier Office of Continuing Medical Education (EOCME) is accredited by the Accreditation Council for Continuing Medical Education (ACCME) to provide continuing medical education for physicians.

The EOCME designates this enduring material for a maximum of 15 *AMA PRA Category 1 Credit*(s)™. Physicians should claim only the credit commensurate with the extent of their participation in the activity.

All other health care professionals requesting continuing education credit for this enduring material will be issued a certificate of participation.

DISCLOSURE OF CONFLICTS OF INTEREST

The EOCME assesses conflict of interest with its instructors, faculty, planners, and other individuals who are in a position to control the content of CME activities. All relevant conflicts of interest that are identified are thoroughly vetted by EOCME for fair balance, scientific objectivity, and patient care recommendations. EOCME is committed to providing its learners with CME activities that promote improvements or quality in healthcare and not a specific proprietary business or a commercial interest.

The planning committee, staff, authors and editors listed below have identified no financial relationships or relationships to products or devices they or their spouse/life partner have with commercial interest related to the content of this CME activity:

Prachi P. Agarwal, MBBS, MS; Spencer C. Behr, MD; Maurice B. Bizino, MD; Nicholas S. Burris, MD; Danielle Chan, MD; Pierluigi Ciet, MD; Paul de Heer, MSc; Adam L. Dorfman, MD; Juliano Lara Fernandes, MD, MBA, PhD; Robert Groves, MD; Henrik Haraldsson, PhD; Kristen Helm; Charles B. Higgins, MD; Michael D. Hope, MD; Brynne Hunter; Masaki Ishida, MD; Kimberly Kallianos, MD; Nazima N. Kathiria, DO; Suma H. Konety, MD, MS; Hildebrandus J. Lamb, MD, PhD; Sandy Lavery; Diana E. Litmanovich, MD; Jing Liu, PhD; Maria Clara N. Lorca, MD; Jimmy C. Lu, MD; Maryam Ghadimi Mahani, MD; Carolina Masri, MD; Gustavo L. Moraes, MD; Suresh K. Mukherji, MD, MBA, FACR; David M. Naeger, MD; Karen G. Ordovas, MD, MAS; Carlos Eduardo Rochitte, MD, PhD; Albert de Roos, MD, PhD; Hajime Sakuma, MD; Michael L. Sala, MD; David Saloner, PhD; Jan W.A. Smit, MD, PhD; Brandon M. Smith, MD; Lynne S. Steinbach, MD, FACR; Karthikeyan Subramaniam; Ashenafi M. Tamene, MD; Shawn D. Teague, MD; Pieternel van der Tol, MSc; John Vassallo; Andrew G. Webb, PhD; Marianna Zagurovskaya, MD; Stefan L. Zimmerman, MD.

The planning committee, staff, authors and editors listed below have identified financial relationships or relationships to products or devices they or their spouse/life partner have with commercial interest related to the content of this CME activity:

UNAPPROVED/OFF-LABEL USE DISCLOSURE

The EOCME requires CME faculty to disclose to the participants:
1. When products or procedures being discussed are off-label, unlabelled, experimental, and/or investigational (not US Food and Drug Administration [FDA] approved); and
2. Any limitations on the information presented, such as data that are preliminary or that represent ongoing research, interim analyses, and/or unsupported opinions. Faculty may discuss information about pharmaceutical agents that is outside of FDA-approved labelling. This information is intended solely for CME and is not intended to promote off-label use of these medications. If you have any questions, contact the medical affairs department of the manufacturer for the most recent prescribing information.

TO ENROLL

To enroll in the *Magnetic Resonance Imaging Clinics of North America* Continuing Medical Education program, call customer service at 1-800-654-2452 or sign up online at http://www.theclinics.com/home/cme. The CME program is available to subscribers for an additional annual fee of USD 250.

METHOD OF PARTICIPATION

In order to claim credit, participants must complete the following:

1. Complete enrolment as indicated above.
2. Read the activity.
3. Complete the CME Test and Evaluation. Participants must achieve a score of 70% on the test. All CME Tests and Evaluations must be completed online.

CME INQUIRIES/SPECIAL NEEDS

For all CME inquiries or special needs, please contact elsevierCME@elsevier.com.

Foreword
Cardiac Imaging

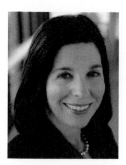

Lynne S. Steinbach, MD, FACR
Consulting Editor

This issue of *Magnetic Resonance Imaging Clinics of North America* focuses on Cardiac MR imaging, a very critical and rapidly evolving field. It is extremely important for those who are performing and interpreting these studies to stay current with the latest advances as well as to review the subject in a comprehensive manner.

My esteemed colleague at the University of California–San Francisco, Professor Karen Ordovas, as editor of this issue, has assembled an excellent volume that delivers comprehensive, up-to-date information about this discipline. The authors are from various institutions at the forefront of cardiac MR imaging around the world. These include University of Washington, Beth Israel Deaconess Medical Center, University of Indiana, Jose Michel Kalaf Research Institute in Brazil, Johns Hopkins, University of Leiden, University of Minnesota, University of Michigan, and the Mie Institution in Japan. These authors discuss current basics and new sequences as well as new modalities, including PET-MR, which is starting to infiltrate the clinical market with its unique capabilities.

Dr Mukherji and I would like to thank Dr Ordovas and the authors of these articles for their excellent contributions to the field of Cardiac MR imaging.

Lynne S. Steinbach, MD, FACR
Department of Radiology and Biomedical Imaging
University of California San Francisco
505 Parnassus
San Francisco, CA 94143-0628, USA

E-mail address:
lynne.steinbach@ucsf.edu

Magn Reson Imaging Clin N Am 23 (2015) xv
http://dx.doi.org/10.1016/j.mric.2014.09.013
1064-9689/15/$ – see front matter

Preface
Updates in Cardiac MRI

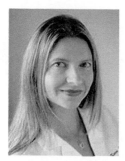

Karen G. Ordovas, MD, MAS
Editor

It is with great enthusiasm that I introduce this issue of the *Magnetic Resonance Imaging Clinics of North America* focused on cardiac MR Imaging. Thanks to the efforts of many world-renowned cardiac imagers, we succeeded in our goal of reviewing topics of great interest to our specialty.

The articles in this publication highlight the current state-of-the-art applications of cardiac MR imaging, with a special emphasis on novel available techniques and clinical indications, including techniques for image acceleration, 4-dimensional flow quantification, tissue characterization, and myocardial strain imaging. We also discuss current developments and their potential future applications and examine the role of cardiac MR imaging as a prognostic biomarker of cardiovascular disease, a growing application in the field and focus of multiple recent clinical trials.

The potential role of PET-MR for cardiac disease assessment is also included, with illustrations of current perspectives and limitations of the use of this combined imaging approach. Cardiac MR imaging applications in oncologic patients and special considerations for imaging female patients are also important topics covered in this publication.

MR imaging of the heart is now an established modality for the evaluation of patients with several cardiac diseases, and guidelines of major professional cardiac societies list it as an important method for diagnosis and follow-up of patients with both congenital and acquired heart diseases. The future of cardiac MR is here! The goal now is to image faster and more efficiently, while understanding where MR better serves our patients and changes the disease outcomes.

By the end of the issue, it is my hope that readers will have an appreciation of the wide range of current clinical applications of cardiac MR as well as an understanding of future applications of the method. Enjoy your reading!

Karen G. Ordovas, MD, MAS
Associate Professor of Radiology
Director of Cardiac Imaging
University of California, San Francisco
505 Parnassus Avenue, M396, Box 0628
San Francisco, CA 94143-0628, USA

E-mail address:
karen.ordovas@ucsf.edu

Magn Reson Imaging Clin N Am 23 (2015) xvii
http://dx.doi.org/10.1016/j.mric.2014.09.012
1064-9689/15/$ – see front matter © 2015 Published by Elsevier Inc.

MR Physics in Practice
How to Optimize Acquisition Quality and Time for Cardiac MR Imaging

David Saloner, PhD[a,b], Jing Liu, PhD[b], Henrik Haraldsson, PhD[a,*]

KEYWORDS

- Motion • Gating • Acceleration • Parallel imaging • Compressed sensing

KEY POINTS

- Cardiac MRI provides images with a variety of tissue contrasts, which can be exploited in the diagnosis of different cardiac conditions.
- A major limitation in cardiac MRI is motion caused by the beating heart and respiration, which further constrains the trade-offs between the image quality and acquisition time.
- Utilization of multiple-channel coils generally provides improved image quality, and higher field strength scanners provide higher signal-to-noise ratio.

INTRODUCTION

Cardiac MRI provides images with a variety of tissue contrasts and this can be exploited in the diagnosis of different cardiac conditions. All of these contrasts require sufficient image quality to provide accurate diagnoses. Image quality in MR is based on the underlying MR physics, and usually requires trade-offs between the signal-to-noise ratio (SNR), spatial resolution, acquisition time, and so on. A major limitation in cardiac MRI is the motion caused by the beating heart and by respiration, which further constrains the trade-offs. The utilization of multiple-channel coils generally provides improved image quality, and higher field strength scanners provide higher SNR. In this paper, we introduce current practical approaches to optimize cardiac MRI quality and scan time. We review motion compensation methods, acceleration techniques, and practical examples for optimizing the image quality and scan time.

CARDIAC AND RESPIRATORY MOTION

Central to cardiac MRI is how to address the cardiac and respiratory motion. These two sources of motion are commonly managed independently to reduce image artifacts.

Cardiac Triggering

Cardiac MR images are typically reconstructed from data acquired over several heart beats. To account for cardiac motion the acquisition is synchronized with the echocardiographic signal. Morphologic, single time frame images are commonly acquired by acquiring multiple data samples during mid diastole when the heart has minimal motion. This allows for a relatively long temporal window with minimal motion artifacts, resulting in a shorter acquisition time. For functional time resolved data, the trade-off between temporal window and the total acquisition time becomes more apparent. A higher temporal resolution

The authors have nothing to disclose.

[a] Department of Radiology and Biomedical Imaging, University of California San Francisco, 505 Parnassus Avenue, San Francisco, CA 94143-0628, USA; [b] Department of Veterans Affairs Medical Center, 4150 Clement Street, San Francisco, CA 94121, USA
* Corresponding author. Box 2520, 4150 Clement Street, VAMC Room BA-51, San Francisco, CA 94121.
E-mail address: Henrik.Haraldsson@ucsf.edu

Magn Reson Imaging Clin N Am 23 (2015) 1–6
http://dx.doi.org/10.1016/j.mric.2014.08.004
1064-9689/15/$ – see front matter © 2015 Elsevier Inc. All rights reserved.

requires a narrower temporal window for each time frame, which requires a longer total acquisition time. On the other hand, lowering the temporal resolution widens the temporal window used to reconstruct the images, which makes it more prone to temporal blurring.

Prospective and Retrospective Modes

Time resolved cardiac image can be acquired in two different modes: Prospective or retrospective. In prospective imaging, data acquisition starts at the detection of the echocardiographic trigger and data are acquired for a predefined number of temporal phases, after which the acquisition is idle until the next trigger occurs. The predefined number of temporal phases is prescribed to cover an interval that is slightly shorter than the duration of the cardiac cycle to ensure that the system is ready for the next trigger. If the number of phases is low, the acquisition is limited to the early parts of the cardiac cycle, and if the number is too high, the acquisition may continue into the next cardiac cycle, thereby missing the trigger of that cardiac cycle. Missed triggers result in longer acquisition times. Retrospective acquisition, on the other hand, does not require a predefined number of time frames as the data are sorted after they are acquired. Furthermore, retrospective sequences run continuously, without any breaks in data acquisition between cardiac cycles, and the steady state can therefore be preserved.

Respiratory Motion

The heart is located next to the diaphragm, and respiration is therefore a major cause of motion artifacts in cardiac MRI. Analogous to cardiac motion, the remedy for respiratory motion is to acquire data at certain stages in the respiratory cycle. This can be achieved by breath-holds, navigator gating, or pneumatic bellows triggering.

Breath-hold methods are a simple and reliable means to minimize respiratory motion as long as the acquisition time is sufficiently short. However, patients often find even short breath-holds challenging. Furthermore, to cover an image volume, multiple breath-holds are usually required, which may result in slice misregistration error owing to the difficulty in consistently reproducing the same breath-hold position. To obtain short breath-holds, the breath-hold duration can be reduced using acceleration techniques described herein.

Navigator gating is a suitable option for sequences that require longer acquisition time. In navigated sequences, a separate readout is introduced to detect the movement of the diaphragm. A threshold is set for the maximum allowable excursion of the diaphragm through the acquisition, and data acquired outside that threshold are rejected and reacquired when the diaphragm returns back within the threshold. A narrow acceptance window therefore reduces the extent to which respiration degrades image quality, but increases total acquisition time. Navigator gating is a relatively accurate method for tracking respiratory motion, because it measures the actual displacement of the diaphragm. However, it continuously interrupts data acquisition, which breaks the steady state of the readout and may result in artifacts.

ACCELERATION

Compared with other medical imaging modalities such as ultrasonography and computed tomography, MR imaging is relatively time consuming, resulting in patient discomfort, motion-related artifacts, or limitations of imaging capabilities. The speed of the acquisition is fundamentally limited by physical and physiologic constrains. The most common approach used to accelerate the acquisition is therefore to reduce the amount of data acquired to reconstruct an image. However, the missing information that results from data undersampling causes artifacts in the reconstructed image. The goal of different acceleration methods is therefore to recover images with minimal artifacts, even in the presence of undersampled data.

Partial Acquisition and Non-Cartesian Acquisition

Most of the image energy is concentrated around the low frequency k-space center, whereas the high-frequency outer k-space contains less visual information. This can be exploited to reduce the acquisition time. One commonly used method is partial Fourier acquisition, which takes advantage of the symmetry properties of k-space. In this method, only one half of k-space is fully sampled in the phase or the slice encoding direction.[1] With this method, nearly 50% of k-space need not be explicitly acquired but can be mathematically reconstructed, correspondingly reducing the total acquisition time. Instead of sampling the data uniformly, non-Cartesian acquisitions such as spiral and radial sampling can be designed to accelerate scan time by undersampling the outer portions of k-space and sufficiently or overly sampling the central k-space.[2,3]

Sliding Window, Keyhole, Time-Resolved Imaging of Contrast Kinetics

For dynamic imaging with multiple time frames, the data can be undersampled by exploiting

No acceleration   R=2   GRAPPA   R=6
                                          R=4

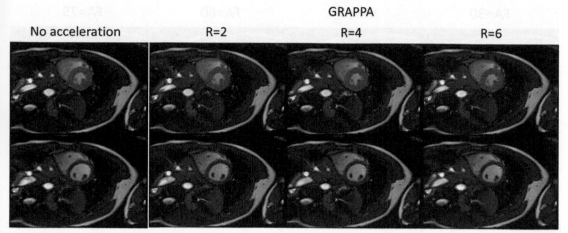

Fig. 1. Parallel imaging acceleration can be used to reduce the acquisition time. Short axis views at end-systolic (*top row*) and end-diastolic (*bottom row*) phases can be seen for different acceleration factors using generalized autocalibrating partially parallel acquisitions (GRAPPA). Notice the decreased signal-to-noise ratio (SNR) with increased acceleration factor.

redundancies in the temporal domain, generally called as k–t methods. View sharing is a commonly used method to accelerate time-resolved acquisitions.[4–6] The k-space is interleaved into multiple segments, and the time frames are reconstructed by sharing data with adjacent time frames. Usually, the k-space center is acquired at each time frame and the high frequencies are interleaved. The fully sampled high-frequency data are combined from all the time frames and shared for all the frames.

Parallel Imaging

Each coil element in a multiple receiver coil has its unique spatial location, and when combined that data contain spatial redundancies. In parallel imaging these spatial redundancies are exploited to reconstruct images from undersampled data. In theory, the greatest acceleration factor that can be achieved is of the order of the number of the coil elements. In practice, the SNR loss related to the parallel acquisition often limits the

vps=10, 10s   vps=20, 6s   vps=40, 4s   vps=60, 4s

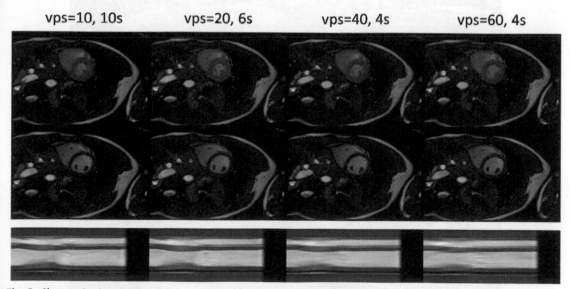

Fig. 2. Short axis view images at end-systolic (*first row*) and end-diastolic (*second row*) phases with different selections of views per segment (10, 20, 40, and 60). The *third row* show a cross-section profile (a *vertical line* in the short axis view image) plotted along time (*horizontal axis*). Notice the increased temporal blurring (horizontally in the *third row*) with increased views per segment.

FA=30   FA=45   FA=60   FA=75

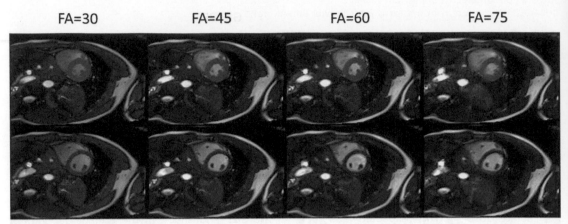

Fig. 3. Short axis images acquired with different flip angles (FA). The *top row* shows the images at end-systolic phase, and the *bottom row* shows the end-diastolic phase. Different signal-to-noise ratio (SNR) and contrast are seen for the different flip angles.

achievable acceleration factor. Clinically used parallel imaging methods include sensitivity encoding for fast MRI (SENSE) and generalized autocalibrating partially parallel acquisitions (GRAPPA),[7,8] which have various names depending on the vendors. Parallel imaging also allows combination with k–t methods.[9,10]

Compressed Sensing

Recently, the compressed sensing technique has been introduced into the field of MRI to achieve scan time acceleration by recovering images with undersampled data.[11] Compression techniques are commonly used in applications such as MP3 audios and JPG images. Similarly, under certain constraints, the MR images can be compressed with specific transformations and can be represented by a small portion of the data. This permits the user to acquire less data (shorter scan time) but maintain sufficient image quality. Furthermore, the compressed sensing technique can also be combined with parallel imaging and k–t techniques, achieving high acceleration factors.[12,13]

True FISP   GRE

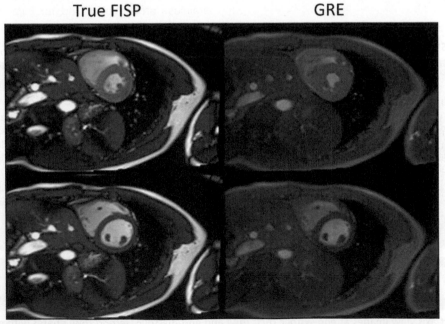

Fig. 4. Images acquired with TrueFISP and GRE. The TrueFISP acquisition provides a greater signal-to-noise ratio (SNR). *Black bands* are present in the arm in the lower right corner in the TrueFISP acquisition, but are located outside the region of interest.

2.7×2.7×6.0mm　　2.0×2.0×6.0mm　　1.3×1.3×6.0mm　　2.0×2.0×3.0mm

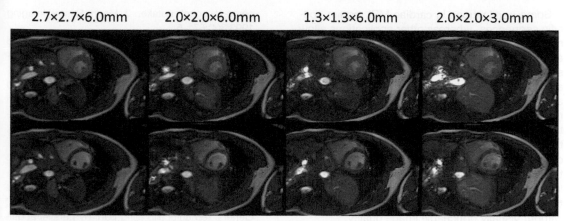

Fig. 5. Images acquired with various spatial resolutions. Reduced spatial resolution increases the signal-to-noise ratio (SNR), which can be traded for a shortened acquisition time.

PRACTICAL EXAMINATIONS FOR OPTIMIZING IMAGE QUALITY AND SCAN TIME

Practical examination implementations achieve a trade-off between image quality and scan time. In this section, we describe examples of practical examinations to explain the relationships between the scan parameters and introduce how the trade-off between the image quality and scan time can be optimized.

Parallel imaging is an efficient way to reduce scan time, but sacrifices the SNR, and may introduce technique depended artifacts. **Fig. 1** shows data from accelerated acquisitions using GRAPPA, for which the end-systolic and diastolic phases are shown.

By modifying the number of k-space lines per segments per view the acquisition time can be reduced at the expense of the temporal resolution. In **Fig. 2**, the number of views per segment varies, ranging between 10 and 60. The reconstructed number of cardiac phases was chosen to be the same by applying sliding window to share the data among different cardiac phases.

The flip angle influence both SNR and contrast of the blood and myocardium in the cardiac image. In **Fig. 3**, data were acquire with different flip angles. The measured SNRs of the blood in the left ventricles were 3.9, 5.2, 4.8, and 2.8 for flip angles of 30°, 45°, 60°, and 75° respectively, and the corresponding contrast-to-noise ratio between blood and myocardium were 3.9, 5.1, 4.8, and 2.7. It suggests a flip angle of 45° to 60° could be chosen to achieve the optimal blood SNR and blood-to-myocardium contrast-to-noise ratio.

Full　　　　　Fourier 6/8　　　　　Fourier 4/8

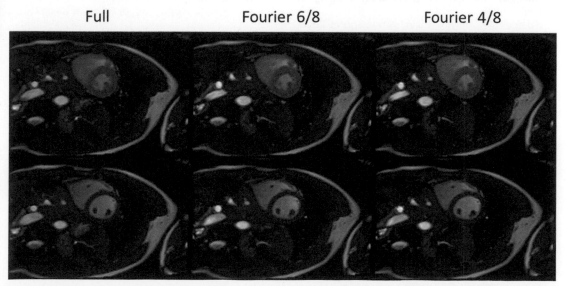

Fig. 6. Partial phase encoding can be chosen to reduce scan time while maintaining image quality.

Some applications in cardiac MRI require specific sequences, whereas other applications allow multiple choices. The choice does in these cases affect many aspects of the image quality. **Fig. 4** show images acquired with TrueFISP and GRE, and illustrates the differences in SNR, contrast, and technique specific artifacts. Reduced spatial resolution increases the SNR, which could be traded for a shorter acquisition time. **Fig. 5** shows the trade-off between images acquired with different image spatial resolutions. Partial acquisition can be used to shorten the acquisition time or increase the temporal resolution. In **Fig. 6** the scan time was reduced by partial phase encodings without visually noticeable image quality.

ACKNOWLEDGMENTS

Funding support was provided by a VA MERIT Review grant (DS), and grant K25EB014914 from the NIH (JL).

REFERENCES

1. Noll DC, Nishimura DG, Macovski A. Homodyne detection in magnetic resonance imaging. IEEE Trans Med Imaging 1991;10(2):154–63. http://dx.doi.org/10.1109/42.79473.
2. Peters DC, Korosec FR, Grist TM, et al. Undersampled projection reconstruction applied to MR angiography. Magn Reson Med 2000;43(1):91–101.
3. Ahn CB, Kim JH, Cho ZH. High-speed spiral-scan echo planar NMR imaging-I. IEEE Trans Med Imaging 1986;5(1):2–7. http://dx.doi.org/10.1109/TMI.1986.4307732.
4. van Vaals JJ, Brummer ME, Dixon WT, et al. "Keyhole" method for accelerating imaging of contrast agent uptake. J Magn Reson Imaging 1993;3(4):671–5.
5. Korosec FR, Frayne R, Grist TM, et al. Time-resolved contrast-enhanced 3D MR angiography. Magn Reson Med 1996;36(3):345–51.
6. Foo TK, Bernstein MA, Aisen AM, et al. Improved ejection fraction and flow velocity estimates with use of view sharing and uniform repetition time excitation with fast cardiac techniques. Radiology 1995;195(2):471–8.
7. Pruessmann KP, Weiger M, Scheidegger MB, et al. SENSE: sensitivity encoding for fast MRI. Magn Reson Med 1999;42(5):952–62.
8. Griswold MA, Jakob PM, Heidemann RM, et al. Generalized autocalibrating partially parallel acquisitions (GRAPPA). Magn Reson Med 2002;47(6):1202–10.
9. Kozerke S, Tsao J, Razavi R, et al. Accelerating cardiac cine 3D imaging using k-t BLAST. Magn Reson Med 2004;52(1):19–26.
10. Tsao J, Boesiger P, Pruessmann KP. k-t BLAST and k-t SENSE: dynamic MRI with high frame rate exploiting spatiotemporal correlations. Magn Reson Med 2003;50(5):1031–42.
11. Lustig M, Donoho D, Pauly JM. Sparse MRI: the application of compressed sensing for rapid MR imaging. Magn Reson Med 2007;58(6):1182–95. http://dx.doi.org/10.1002/mrm.21391.
12. Otazo R, Kim D, Axel L, et al. Combination of compressed sensing and parallel imaging for highly accelerated first-pass cardiac perfusion MRI. Magn Reson Med 2010;64(3):767–76. http://dx.doi.org/10.1002/mrm.22463.
13. Usman M, Prieto C, Schaeffter T, et al. k-t group sparse: a method for accelerating dynamic MRI. Magn Reson Med 2011. http://dx.doi.org/10.1002/mrm.22883.

Ventricular Mechanics
Techniques and Applications

Maria Clara N. Lorca, MD, Henrik Haraldsson, PhD, Karen G. Ordovas, MD, MAS*

KEYWORDS

- Strain • Magnetic resonance • Cardiac • Imaging • Ventricular mechanics

KEY POINTS

- Regional function of the myocardium can be quantified using myocardial strain analysis.
- Myocardial strain is defined as the relative lengthening of the tissue, thus: a normalized measure of deformation.
- The main parameters used to quantify strain on magnetic resonance imaging are circumferential, longitudinal, and radial strain.
- Many cardiac magnetic resonance techniques have been developed for detection and quantification of regional strain abnormalities including steady-state free-precession cine, tagging, and displacement encoding with stimulated echoes.
- Recent clinical studies have shown potential use of these techniques for risk stratification and treatment guidance in patients with congenital and acquired heart diseases.

INTRODUCTION

Many cardiac diseases do not affect the heart globally in an early stage.[1] Normal global measures such as ejection fraction can therefore be insensitive to these early regional dysfunctions.[2] Thus, the assessment of the regional myocardium function with magnetic resonance imaging (MRI) poses as a novel potentially important tool for early identification of cardiac pathology.

Regional function of the myocardium can be quantified using myocardial strain analysis. Myocardial strain is defined as the relative lengthening of the tissue, thus: a normalized measure of deformation.[3,4] Cardiac MRI (cMRI) is considered the reference standard for measurement of myocardial strain. Some of the cardiac MRI techniques used for measuring regional myocardial functions are myocardial steady-state free precession (SSFP) cine, tagging, displacement encoding with stimulated echoes (DENSE),[1] strain encoding imaging (SENC), and feature tracking techniques.[2]

From a biomechanical point of view, it would be preferable to present the strain given the fiber structure of the heart; however, the complex geometry of the heart makes this challenging. Therefore, the main parameters used to quantify strain on MRI are circumferential, longitudinal, and radial strain (**Fig. 1**). Another measure used to describe deformation is strain rate, which describes the rate at which the strain is changing over time.[5] Finally, it is possible to quantify diastolic function based on myocardial strain. The main parameter used for quantification of diastolic function is the strain relaxation index (SRI), which is calculated based on the relationship of the circumferential strain with strain rate curves.[6]

TECHNIQUES
Steady-State Free Precession Cine

SSFP has been used routinely in clinical practice for quantification of regional myocardial function. Qualitatively, this technique allows for visual

The authors have nothing to disclose.

Department of Radiology and Biomedical Imaging, University of California San Francisco, 505 Parnassus Avenue, Box 0628, San Francisco, CA 94143, USA

* Corresponding author.

E-mail address: Karen.ordovas@ucsf.edu

Magn Reson Imaging Clin N Am 23 (2015) 7–13

http://dx.doi.org/10.1016/j.mric.2014.08.005

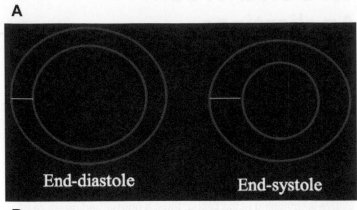

A

End-diastole   End-systole

Fig. 1. Parameters for cardiac strain quantification. Diagrams illustrate measurements as changes in distance between 2 points aligned to the transmural myocardial axis for radial strain (A), aligned to the circumference of the heart for circumferential strain (B), and aligned to the long axis of the heart for longitudinal strain (C).

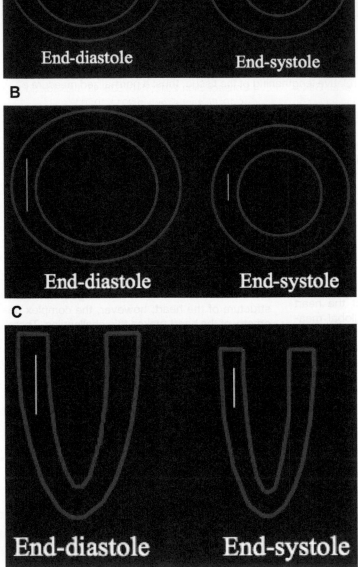

B

End-diastole   End-systole

C

End-diastole   End-systole

inspection of myocardial thickening during the cardiac cycle in all cardiac regions. Common cardiac planes, named short axis, horizontal long axis, and vertical long axis, provide comprehensive assessment of myocardial contractility in the anterior, lateral, inferior, and septal regions, including the apex, midventricular level, and base of the heart.

In addition to visual assessment of cardiac contractility, postprocessing tools allow for quantification of myocardial thickening during the cardiac cycle, which consists of the increase in myocardial wall thickness from end-diastole to end-systole, and is expressed in millimeters. Measurement of wall thickening in the short-axis plane corresponds to the radial strain measurement of the entire transmural myocardium, and can be obtained in each of the 16 American Heart Association (AHA) cardiac segments.

Tagging

Tagging is a cardiac magnetic resonance technique introduced by Zerhouni and colleagues[7] that noninvasively creates markers in the moving tissue in order to observe and assess myocardial motion. Tagging creates visible orthogonal saturation lines (by perturbing the magnetization) that can be imaged and tracked (**Fig. 2**).[2] Because magnetization is an intrinsic property of the underlying tissue, the tagged lines follow tissue movement, therefore allowing for measurement of the deformation. The main techniques used for strain measurement with tagged lines are based on spatial modulation of magnetization (SPAMM).[2,8]

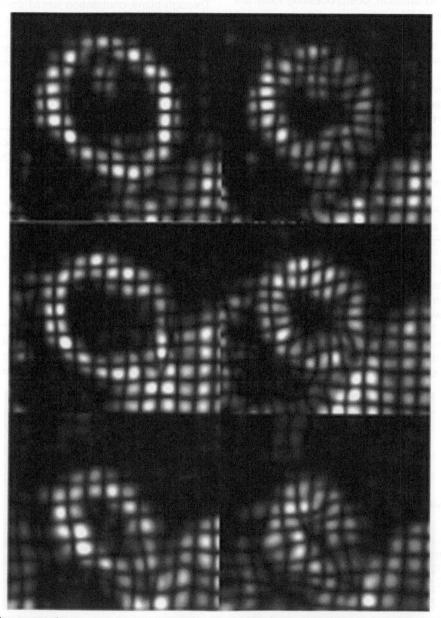

Fig. 2. Tagging magnetic resonance images acquired at the basilar (*top*), midventricular (*middle*), and apical (*bottom*) levels, during end-diastole (*left*) and end-systole (*right*). Note the distortion of the vertical and horizontal tags during the cardiac cycle in this patient after repair of tetralogy of Fallot. (*From* Ordovas KG, Carlsson M, Lease KE, et al. Impaired regional left ventricular strain after repair of tetralogy of Fallot. J Magn Reson Imaging 2012;35(1):79–85; with permission.)

This technique has been further developed to reduce the fading of the tag lines fading at end-diastole using complementary SPAMM (CSPAMM). The main advantage of this method is its extensive validation studies, including animal and clinical studies.[9–12] In addition, a range of normal values has already been determined. Disadvantages of the method are mainly related to the fact that the tagged lines fade over time and may not be clearly detected at the end of the cardiac cycle. In addition, postprocessing tools are available, but the process is very time consuming. In addition to conventional tag analysis techniques, a method of extracting myocardial strain measurement from tagging sequences utilizing the tagging frequency called harmonic phase is widely used, and is currently considered the most reliable and reproducible method for postprocessing of tagged images.[13–15]

Displacement Encoding with Stimulated Echoes

Displacement encoding with stimulated echoes (DENSE) is an alternative method to assess cardiac motion with MRI. Tissue displacement is measured at the pixel level, providing both in-plane and through-plane motion, and it can be performed in a 2-dimensional or 3-dimensional fashion. In this technique, there are no visual tagged lines generated, but instead the tracking is based on the differences in phase of the MRI signal between the stationary and the moving spins (**Fig. 3**). The main advantages of this technique are in its high spatial resolution, its inherent black blood, which simplifies the delineation of the myocardium, and easy postprocessing

analysis. Disadvantages of the method are related to the lack of extensive clinical research validating its applications.

Strain-encoding Imaging

Strain encoding imaging (SENC) is another technique that can be used for measuring myocardial strain. SENC does this by applying out-of-plane tags to modulate the magnetization in the through plane direction with a predefined frequency. Through-plane contraction would cause this frequency to increase, whereas stretch would cause it to decrease. To measure the change of frequency, SENC uses readouts with different through-plane phase encodings, and the frequency is obtained by straightforward calculations of the signal of these different phase encodings.[16]

Feature Tracking

Cardiovascular magnetic resonance feature tracking (FT) is a postprocessing method that detects quantitative wall motion derived from SSFP cine imaging.

FT measures tissue voxel motion and derivation of wall mechanics and strain without the need for acquisition of additional sequences.[17–19]

This feature showed reasonable agreement with tagging and acceptable interobserver reproducibility.[20,21]

CLINICAL APPLICATIONS

The main area of clinical research on strain parameters measured by cardiac MRI has been ischemic heart disease. It has been shown that systolic strain magnetic resonance parameters are

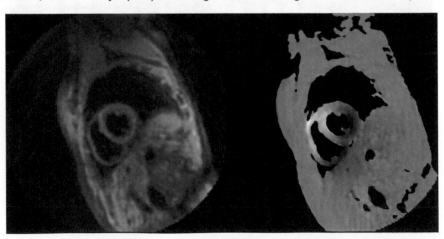

Fig. 3. Displacement encoding with stimulated echoes (DENSE). The magnitude in DENSE MRI depicts the anatomy, as seen to the left, whereas the phase provides information of the displacement, as seen to the right, where the phase is encoded to show displacement left-to-right. The brighter anterioseptal region indicates displacement to the right, while the darker inferiolateral region indicates displacement to the left. The phase data have been masked for illustrative purpose.

strongly associated with known risk factors of coronary artery disease.[22,23] The most important study that evaluated the role of MRI strain imaging as a predictor of heart disease is the CARDIA (Coronary Artery Risk Development in Young Adults) arm of the MESA (Multi-Ethnic Study of Atherosclerosis) trial.[5]

In the CARDIA study, 1768 patients randomly selected from the MESA trial database, which included 6814 men and women without heart disease representing 4 racial/ethnic groups, underwent a tagged MRI at baseline and after 5.5 years of follow-up. Systolic function as measured by circumferential strain was shown to predict incident heart failure and cardiovascular events with a hazard ratio of 1.15 (confidence interval [CI]: 1.01–1.31) after adjustment for known cardiovascular risk factors.[10] An additional study was performed with a subset of the CARDIA study population (743 patients followed for 8 years) to interrogate the role of diastolic dysfunction, measured by SRI calculated from tagged MRI images, as a predictor of incident heart failure and atrial fibrillation.[24] The hazard ratio for SRI was calculated as 2.54 (CI: 1.76–3.66), and remained significant for the combined heart failure and atrial fibrillation end points as well as for heart failure alone after adjustment for common heart failure predictors.

Clinical applications of myocardial strain measurements on MRI in patients with nonischemic cardiac diseases have also been interrogated to a lesser extent. Circumferential left ventricular strain has been shown to be abnormal in patients with arrythmogenic right ventricular dysplasia compared with normal controls.[25] Patients with dilated cardiomyopathy have also been investigated with MR strain analysis. A recent study has shown abnormal peak systolic torsion in 26 patients with dilated cardiomyopathy patients compared with controls.[26] It has also been shown that circumferential strain improves after partial left ventriculotomy in patients with dilated cardiomyopathy, despite small improvement in global left ventricular (LV) function.[27] Therefore, magnetic resonance strain analysis has the potential to assess efficacy of dilated cardiomyopathy treatments and identify best responders.

Cardiac MRI with myocardial tagging can also help identify early systolic and diastolic dysfunction in hypertrophic cardiomyopathy (HCM) disease, despite normal global functional parameters. Ennis and colleagues[23] showed circumferential septal strain and diastolic strain in all regions significantly reduced in patients with HCM and normal LV ejection fraction (LVEF). In addition, tagging was able to identify regional strain abnormalities in areas of nonhypertrophied myocardium of patients with HCM.[26,28] Finally, myocardial tagging can aid in the differentiation between an athlete's heart and asymptomatic nonobstructive hypertrophic cardiomyopathy or hypertensive hypertrophy.[27]

Another potential important application of magnetic strain imaging is for depicting and mapping dyssynchrony in patients with decreased LV function. It has been shown in multiple small single-center trials that the presence of dyssynchrony predicts better response to cardiac resynchronization therapy (CRT), with higher ejection fraction and improvement of symptoms.[14] However, a large multicenter trial using echocardiography for dyssynchrony evaluation (Predictors of Response to CRT [PROSPECT]) failed to demonstrate improved survival rates in patients who had CRT based on documented dyssynchrony, compared with patients without evidence of dyssynchrony prior to treatment.[5] Tagging has the ability to generate precise and reproducible dyssynchrony maps for guidance of CRT.[29] Future clinical trials are needed to assess the role of magnetic resonance tagging for mortality reduction after CRT.

Congenital Heart Disease

Strain imaging has been investigated in patients with congenital heart diseases, particularly tetralogy of Fallot, in an effort to characterize early myocardial dysfunction that could inform the need for pulmonary valve replacement or be a prognostic indicator. Ordovas and colleagues[16] have previously demonstrated decreased circumferential strain in patients with tetralogy of Fallot and preserved global contractility (normal LVEF) compared with normal controls using tagging MRI (Fig. 4). LV dysfunction has been identified as a poor prognostic parameter in patients after repair of tetralogy of Fallot.[21] Therefore, the authors suggested that identification of early subclinical LV dysfunction may be an important clinical parameter to guide early interventions in these patients.[16] In addition, wall thickening is particularly abnormal in the ventricular septum in patients with abnormal septal excursion during the cardiac cycle, an indication that interventricular interaction may play an important role in LV dysfunction after repair of tetralogy of Fallot.[30]

In addition, Wald and colleagues[31] have quantified strain abnormalities of the right ventricular outflow tract using tissue tracking MRI, and have shown that regional abnormalities in the right ventricular outflow tract (RVOT) adversely affect global right ventricular function and exercise capacity after tetralogy of Fallot repair. The authors

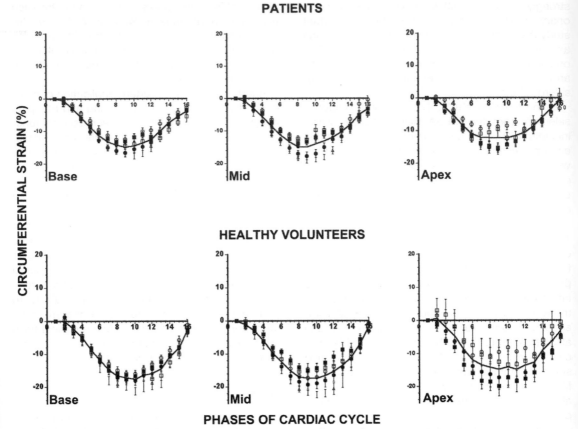

Fig. 4. Mean circumferential strain during the cardiac cycle is shown in the basilar, midventricular, and apical levels of patients (*top*) and healthy volunteers (*bottom*). Note the decreased circumferential strain in the patients compared with normal volunteers. (*From* Ordovas KG, Carlsson M, Lease KE, et al. Impaired regional left ventricular strain after repair of tetralogy of Fallot. J Magn Reson Imaging 2012;35(1):79–85; with permission.)

concluded that these regional measures may have important implications for patient management, including RVOT reconstruction, at the time of pulmonary valve replacement.

SUMMARY

Multiple magnetic resonance methods are available for detection and quantification of myocardial strain abnormalities. Recent clinical studies have shown potential use of these techniques for risk stratification and treatment guidance in patients with congenital and acquired heart diseases, particularly for early detection of heart failure.

REFERENCES

1. Castillo E, Lima JA, Bluemke DA. Regional myocardial function: advances in MR imaging and analysis. Radiographics 2003;23(Spec No):S127–40.
2. Ibrahim el SH. Myocardial tagging by cardiovascular magnetic resonance: evolution of techniques–pulse sequences, analysis algorithms, and applications. J Cardiovasc Magn Reson 2011;13:36.
3. Mirsky I, Parmley WW. Assessment of passive elastic stiffness for isolated heart muscle and the intact heart. Circ Res 1973;33:233–43.
4. Tee M, Noble JA, Bluemke DA. Imaging techniques for cardiac strain and deformation: comparison of echocardiography, cardiac magnetic resonance and cardiac computed tomography. Expert Rev Cardiovasc Ther 2013;11:221–31.
5. Chung ES, Leon AR, Tavazzi L, et al. Results of the Predictors of Response to CRT (PROSPECT) trial. Circulation 2008;117:2608–16.
6. Nickel JC, Fradet Y, Boake RC, et al. Efficacy and safety of finasteride therapy for benign prostatic hyperplasia: results of a 2-year randomized controlled trial (the PROSPECT study). PROscar Safety Plus Efficacy Canadian Two year Study. CMAJ 1996;155:1251–9.
7. Zerhouni EA, Parish DM, Rogers WJ, et al. Human heart: tagging with MR imaging—a method for noninvasive assessment of myocardial motion. Radiology 1988;169:59–63.

8. White JA, Fine N, Gula LJ, et al. Fused whole-heart coronary and myocardial scar imaging using 3-T CMR. Implications for planning of cardiac resynchronization therapy and coronary revascularization. JACC Cardiovasc Imaging 2010;3:921–30.

9. Castillo E, Osman NF, Rosen BD, et al. Quantitative assessment of regional myocardial function with MR-tagging in a multi-center study: interobserver and intraobserver agreement of fast strain analysis with Harmonic Phase (HARP) MRI. J Cardiovasc Magn Reson 2005;7:783–91.

10. Sullivan RM, Murillo J, Gerritse B, et al. Do baseline diastolic echocardiographic parameters predict outcome after resynchronization therapy? Results from the PROSPECT trial. Pacing Clin Electrophysiol 2013;36:214–20.

11. Kraitchman DL, Sampath S, Castillo E, et al. Quantitative ischemia detection during cardiac magnetic resonance stress testing by use of FastHARP. Circulation 2003;107:2025–30.

12. Phatak NS, Maas SA, Veress AI, et al. Strain measurement in the left ventricle during systole with deformable image registration. Med Image Anal 2009;13:354–61.

13. Delgado V, Bax JJ. Assessment of systolic dyssynchrony for cardiac resynchronization therapy is clinically useful. Circulation 2011;123:640–55.

14. Cleland JG, Daubert JC, Erdmann E, et al. The effect of cardiac resynchronization on morbidity and mortality in heart failure. N Engl J Med 2005;352:1539–49.

15. Delgado V, Ng CT. Assessment of left ventricular systolic function in aortic stenosis and prognostic implications. Eur Heart J Cardiovasc Imaging 2012;13:805–7.

16. Ordovas KG, Carlsson M, Lease KE, et al. Impaired regional left ventricular strain after repair of tetralogy of Fallot. J Magn Reson Imaging 2012;35:79–85.

17. Schuster A, Morton G, Hussain ST, et al. The intraobserver reproducibility of cardiovascular magnetic resonance myocardial feature tracking strain assessment is independent of field strength. Eur J Radiol 2013;82:296–301.

18. Schuster A, Paul M, Bettencourt N, et al. Cardiovascular magnetic resonance myocardial feature tracking for quantitative viability assessment in ischemic cardiomyopathy. Int J Cardiol 2013;166:413–20.

19. Morton G, Schuster A, Jogiya R, et al. Inter-study reproducibility of cardiovascular magnetic resonance myocardial feature tracking. J Cardiovasc Magn Reson 2012;14:43.

20. Augustine D, Lewandowski AJ, Lazdam M, et al. Global and regional left ventricular myocardial deformation measures by magnetic resonance feature tracking in healthy volunteers: comparison with tagging and relevance of gender. J Cardiovasc Magn Reson 2013;15:8.

21. Ghai A, Silversides C, Harris L, et al. Left ventricular dysfunction is a risk factor for sudden cardiac death in adults late after repair of tetralogy of Fallot. J Am Coll Cardiol 2002;40:1675–80.

22. Edvardsen T, Rosen BD, Pan L, et al. Regional diastolic dysfunction in individuals with left ventricular hypertrophy measured by tagged magnetic resonance imaging—the Multi-Ethnic Study of Atherosclerosis (MESA). Am Heart J 2006;151:109–14.

23. Ennis DB, Epstein FH, Kellman P, et al. Assessment of regional systolic and diastolic dysfunction in familial hypertrophic cardiomyopathy using MR tagging. Magn Reson Med 2003;50:638–42.

24. Ambale-Venkatesh B, Armstrong AC, Liu CY, et al. Diastolic function assessed from tagged MRI predicts heart failure and atrial fibrillation over an 8-year follow-up period: the multi-ethnic study of atherosclerosis. Eur Heart J Cardiovasc Imaging 2013;15(4):442–9.

25. Jain A, Shehata ML, Stuber M, et al. Prevalence of left ventricular regional dysfunction in arrhythmogenic right ventricular dysplasia: a tagged MRI study. Circ Cardiovasc Imaging 2010;3:290–7.

26. Maier SE, Fischer SE, McKinnon GC, et al. Evaluation of left ventricular segmental wall motion in hypertrophic cardiomyopathy with myocardial tagging. Circulation 1992;86:1919–28.

27. Jeung MY, Germain P, Croisille P, et al. Myocardial tagging with MR imaging: overview of normal and pathologic findings. Radiographics 2012;32:1381–98.

28. Mishiro Y, Oki T, Iuchi A, et al. Regional left ventricular myocardial contraction abnormalities and asynchrony in patients with hypertrophic cardiomyopathy evaluated by magnetic resonance spatial modulation of magnetization myocardial tagging. Jpn Circ J 1999;63:442–6.

29. Heydari B, Jerosch-Herold M, Kwong RY. Imaging for planning of cardiac resynchronization therapy. JACC Cardiovasc Imaging 2012;5:93–110.

30. Muzzarelli S, Ordovas KG, Cannavale G, et al. Tetralogy of Fallot: impact of the excursion of the interventricular septum on left ventricular systolic function and fibrosis after surgical repair. Radiology 2011;259:375–83.

31. Wald RM, Haber I, Wald R, et al. Effects of regional dysfunction and late gadolinium enhancement on global right ventricular function and exercise capacity in patients with repaired tetralogy of Fallot. Circulation 2009;119:1370–7.

4D Flow MRI Applications for Aortic Disease

Nicholas S. Burris, MD, Michael D. Hope, MD*

KEYWORDS

- 4D flow • Aorta • Aortic aneurysm • Bicuspid aortic valve • Hemodynamic imaging
- Phase contrast MRI • Flow imaging

KEY POINTS

- Three-directional phase contrast MRI (4D flow MRI) is able to visualize and quantify abnormal flow related to a wide variety of aortic pathologies.
- Limitations of the technique, including scan time and artifacts, have been greatly reduced making 4D flow a clinically feasible technique.
- Novel quantitative hemodynamic markers have been developed to characterize abnormal flow, and to investigate underlying mechanisms of disease.
- Markers beyond aortic diameter could improve risk stratification of patients with aortic disease and better determine the timing of intervention.
- Larger, prospective studies are needed to validate the clinical relevance of 4D flow.

OVERVIEW OF AORTIC IMAGING

Aortic disease is a broad term that encompasses related and sometimes overlapping conditions associated with substantial morbidity and mortality, including aortic aneurysm and dissection.[1,2] Imaging has long been used to diagnose and monitor these processes, and along with advances in surgical technique, has markedly improved mortality over the last 50 years.[3] Advances in MRI have led to a more sophisticated understanding of intrinsic and valve-related aortic pathology. These developments not only provide insight into underlying pathophysiology, but also may allow imaging to better predict disease progression and inform the timing of interventions.

Hemodynamic imaging with MRI is among the most recent advances in aortic evaluation. The hemodynamic environment of the aorta is unique with extreme pressure variations, high flow rates, and complex flow patterns that exist in both normal and pathologic states. Phase contrast MRI (PC-MRI) has been utilized in routine conventional cardiac MRI for more than 2 decades to accurately measure these flow dynamics. However, the recent optimization of volumetric, time-resolved (cine) and 3-directional PC-MRI (4D Flow), has led to striking visualization of dynamic flow patterns and quantification of associated abnormal hemodynamics.

In this article, we briefly review common clinical applications of 2-directional (2D) PC-MRI, and discuss the emerging applications of 4D Flow for the thoracic aorta. We aim to highlight ongoing research in the field of aortic 4D Flow imaging by focusing on promising quantitative hemodynamic markers of aortic disease.

Funding: Covidien/Radiological Society of North America Research Scholar Grant RSCH1215 (M.D. Hope).
Disclosures: No conflicts to disclose.
Department of Radiology and Biomedical Imaging, University of California, San Francisco, 505 Parnassus Avenue, Box 0628, San Francisco, CA 94143-0628, USA
* Corresponding author.
E-mail address: michael.hope@ucsf.edu

Magn Reson Imaging Clin N Am 23 (2015) 15–23
http://dx.doi.org/10.1016/j.mric.2014.08.006
1064-9689/15/$ – see front matter © 2015 Elsevier Inc. All rights reserved.

CURRENT CLINICAL 2-DIRECTIONAL FLOW APPLICATIONS

Aortic blood flow imaging with MRI is conventionally performed in 2 dimensions (2D). This means that single-directional velocity data is captured with PC-MRI through or parallel to a prescribed imaging plane. In contrast, 4D Flow imaging captures 3-directional (3D) velocity data through a volume on interest. Currently, conventional 2D evaluation is routinely used in several clinical scenarios: aortic valve disease, cardiac shunt lesions and aortic coarctation.

Echocardiography is commonly used for assessing aortic valvular disease. However, over the past decade, MRI has become increasingly popular because it provides several distinct advantages, including better evaluation of the ascending aorta, more reproducible measurements of regurgitation fraction, and quantitative measurement left ventricular size, function, and mass.[4,5] For evaluation of aortic stenosis, transvalvular gradient is a key parameter for determining disease severity and need for intervention. Transvalvular gradient can be estimated with 2D PC-MRI by imaging parallel the aortic centerline, just beyond the valve, to determine peak jet velocity, which can then be used for estimation of the pressure gradient using the modified Bernoulli equation. However, low temporal resolution and suboptimal imaging plane placement can lead to underestimation of true pressure gradients. For aortic regurgitation, measurement of forward and backward flow volume through the ascending aorta can be used to calculate the regurgitant fraction. Conventional 2D PC-MRI can also be used to quantify cardiac shunt fractions and to assess the hemodynamic impact of aortic coarctation. Similar to aortic regurgitation, through plane flow volumes are measured in the aorta and main pulmonary artery, and the shunt ratio or Qp/Qs can be calculated. In the case of coarctation, acquisition planes are placed across the aorta just distal to the coarctation and at the diaphragm to quantify collateral flow through intercostal vessels, which increases with worsening coarctation severity.[6]

4-DIRECTIONAL FLOW

Multidimensional MRI (eg, 4D Flow) has become an increasingly popular research tool over the past decade. There are several advantages compared with conventional 2D PC sequences: Free breathing, acquisition of 3D velocity data, no need for prospective 2D plane placement, and powerful flow visualization and quantification software. Currently, the main disadvantages of 4D Flow are the need for labor-intensive data after processing, greater susceptibility to motion artifacts, and longer scan times, although scan times have improved dramatically over the last 5 years.

Data Acquisition, Reconstruction, and Fidelity

4D Flow datasets are acquired over multiple cardiac cycles: Using electrocardiographic gating, data are collected over many hundreds of heartbeats and then compiled to create a cine image of a complete, representative cardiac cycle. Without the use of scan acceleration techniques, datasets can take 1 hour to fully acquire, a prohibitively long time for routine applications. When clinical patients are considered, rather than a population of healthy research volunteers, scan time becomes a dominant concern. A significant amount of research effort has been dedicated to reducing 4D Flow scan times, with promising results reported using spiral (rather than conventional Cartesian) acquisitions and data undersampling techniques for acceleration, including compressed sensing. Many studies report scan times of less than 15 minutes, with some groups acquiring data in as few as 5 minutes.[7,8] Data errors with PC-MRI acquisitions have been reported,[9] but can be minimized by routine correction of eddy currents, gradient fields, and Maxwell phase effects.

Data fidelity is an important consideration because 4D Flow data are subject to multiple artifacts. In addition to the technical issues listed, there are other sources of error related to acquisitions spanning numerous heart beats and the presence of underlying pathologic flow characteristics (eg, turbulence, helicity). Confirmation of 4D Flow data fidelity has largely relied on in vitro, in silico, and animal models.[10,11] One in vivo approach for data verification relies on the pathline technique of flow visualization. Pathlines tend to be sensitive to artifact accumulation, because they are calculated by integration over time. Applying conservation-of-mass principles in a specific region of interest, pathlines can be used for data quality verification. Another metric for internal data quality control relies in measurement of aortic (Qs) and pulmonary (Qp) flow rates, which should be equal in the absence of shunts, and can help in the identification of erroneous data. Of note, several important flow parameters are relative to other internal measurements (eg, Qp/Qs, collateral flow, flow displacement) so that the absolute values of the velocity data are less important than relative internal consistency.

Flow Visualization

Several approaches can be used for 4D Flow data visualization, including vector plots and particle traces (ie, streamlines and pathlines), which are typically color coded for velocity data.[12] Whereas a vector plot represents the actual velocity data at a given moment in time, streamlines are imaginary lines that smoothly connect together these vectors for a depiction of an instantaneous flow field. They are visually appealing, but do not represent actual blood flow because they only reflect 1 time point. Pathlines, on the other hand, do represent blood flow through time. They are calculated by releasing imaginary particles into the flow field and then using the dataset to determine where particles will travel in an iterative process through the cardiac cycle. Despite the need for time-intensive post processing, these visualization methods have shown promise for several potential clinical applications, including investigation of valve-related abnormal flow patterns,[13] blood compartmentalization in the ventricles,[14] intimal entry tears and flow patterns in chronic dissection,[15] corrected postrepair flow patterns,[16] and identification of embolic pathways.[17]

QUANTITATIVE HEMODYNAMIC MARKERS

Dynamic flow visualization is an obvious appeal of 4D Flow. It affords an intuitive representation of flow and a qualitative assessment of abnormal flow patterns. Quantitative markers, however, can be derived from 4D Flow datasets to more precisely characterize the hemodynamic consequences of pathologic flow disturbances. Although the true clinical utility of aortic 4D Flow remains to be determined, the ability to measure a diverse set of novel hemodynamic markers is likely to be its most clinically applicable feature.

Clinical guidelines for the management of aortic disease use maximal diameter to risk stratify patients and to set thresholds for operative intervention. Aortic dissection and increased mortality, however, are reported with normal-sized and mildly dilated aortas.[18] The topic of disease progression and aortic diameter is particularly problematic for patients with bicuspid aortic valves (BAV), with marked variability in management reported in routine surgical practice.[19] Markers beyond aortic dimension that reflect the degree of an individual's risk would be useful to better anticipate disease progression and complication. Herein we review promising new flow-related markers in 3 general contexts: Aortic valve disease, valve-related aortic disease, and aortic wall disease.

Aortic Valve Disease

Flow assessment has long been central to the clinical evaluation of the aortic valve. Three main flow-derived parameters are currently measured to determine the severity of aortic stenosis and guide surgical intervention: Transvalvular gradient, valve area, and peak velocity. Although these measurements generally perform well as markers of aortic disease severity, they are not always accurate. For example, gradient estimates using the modified Bernoulli equation do not take into account pressure recovery, and severe aortic stenosis with a low ejection fraction can have low gradients (ie, low-flow/low-gradient severe aortic stenosis).[20,21] A more accurate composite measurement of the increased overall ventricular workload, "valvuloarterial impedance," has been developed, and takes into account the degree of valve obstruction, the ventricular response, and the systemic vascular impedance.[22] Valvuloarterial impedance may better represent the pathologic burden placed on the left ventricle that leads to overload and failure.[20,23]

4D Flow affords a complimentary means of calculating the overall ventricular workload experienced with aortic stenosis. Energy loss can be directly assessed with the technique by 2 recently described methods: Estimation of vicious energy loss and turbulent kinetic energy. Viscous dissipation of energy is a normal feature of aortic flow. For normal laminar flow, it is caused by friction between adjacent fluid layers with different velocities. This friction increases with the abnormal flow features that are seen with aortic valve disease, resulting in substantially elevated viscous energy losses (**Fig. 1**).[24] A limitation of measuring viscous energy loss, however, is that it does not take into account turbulence.

Turbulence is a common feature of post-stenotic flow and a significant contributor to total irreversible pressure loss owing to the dissipation of mechanical energy into heat. Turbulent kinetic energy (TKE) can be estimated with 4D Flow by measuring the distribution of velocities within each imaging voxel: The greater the standard deviation of velocities, the higher the TKE. Recent studies have shown TKE is significantly increased in aortic stenosis, and that TKE measurements by 4D Flow correlate well with established methods of calculating irreversible pressure loss.[25] As a direct imaging measurement of irreversible pressure loss, TKE may best reflect the increased workload placed on the ventricle with aortic stenosis.

Valve-Related Aortic Disease

Valve-related aortic disease has become one of the principal areas of aortic 4D Flow research.

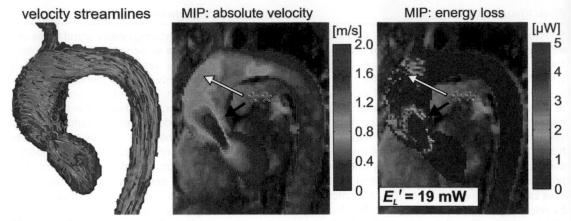

Fig. 1. Systolic velocity streamlines (*left*), maximum intensity projection (MIP) of the 3-dimensinal (3D) velocity field (*middle*), and viscous dissipation (*right*) in the thoracic aorta of a patient with borderline severe stenosis (peak systolic velocity of 4.0 m/s). Regionally high velocity gradients (*double asterisk, black arrow*) result in elevated energy loss. Flow jet impingement at the aortic wall (*double asterisk, white arrow*) is co-located with a region of substantial energy loss. E_L', cumulative peak systolic energy loss in the ascending aorta. (*Courtesy of A. Barker, PhD, and P. van Ooij, PhD, Northwestern University, Chicago, IL.*)

Disease of the aortic valve is frequently associated with abnormal dilation of the ascending aorta (i.e., post-stenotic dilation), especially in the case of congenital BAV. Abnormal hemodynamics and intrinsic aortic wall disease both likely play a role in the development of aortic dilation with BAV, with the relative contribution of each factor debated in the literature.[26] The asymmetry of ascending aortic dilation that is typically seen with BAV, where there is disproportionate dilation of the aortic convexity, suggests an underlying asymmetric driver of disease.[27] 4D Flow research has focused on identifying hemodynamic markers that may be responsible for this dilation pattern and be used to predict disease progression. Research efforts have been invigorated by recent data that shows elevated aortic growth rates with restricted cusp opening angle with BAV, which presumably drives abnormal aortic flow.[28]

Abnormal systolic aortic flow patterns with BAV were first demonstrated with 4D Flow in 2008.[29] Since then, numerous studies have demonstrated similar abnormal flow patterns in the ascending aorta of patients with acquired and congenital aortic valve disease.[30–32] Qualitative visualization of disturbed flow has led to the development of qualitative measures of flow abnormality (**Fig. 2**).

Wall sheer stress (WSS) is an often-reported quantitative marker of abnormal flow. The parameter can be estimated from near-wall velocity gradients with 4D Flow, and represents the frictional force experienced by the endothelium owing to flow viscosity. When deviated from a normal, intermediate range, WSS can adversely affect endothelial activation and signaling. High WSS states have been associated with vascular dilation and remodeling. Using 4D Flow, focally elevated WSS has been demonstrated in patients with BAV at the aortic convexity,[30,33,34] a mechanism that may contribute to asymmetric dilation in this region. Although promising, WSS measurements are challenging. Greater differences between subgroups of patients are demonstrated if peak WSS values are reported,[33] but these peak values are more subject to noise than the mean values that other groups have reported.[34] Furthermore, the accuracy and reliability of WSS estimates derived from 4D Flow data have been called into question, given the difficulty in vessel wall segmentation and limited spatiotemporal resolution.[10,35]

Flow displacement is another quantitative parameter that has shown promise for characterizing BAV-related aortic disease. It measures the displacement of peak systolic flow from the vessel center caused by the presence of a BAV.[36] In the more common BAV leaflet fusion pattern (right–left aortic leaflet fusion [RL]), this displacement is toward the aortic convexity, whereas with the other common fusion (right–noncoronary leaflet fusion [RN]), the displacement is typically more posterior. In some cases, differences in the direction of flow displacement result in completely different orientations of helical flow with RL versus RN fusions (**Fig. 3**). Intriguingly, the differences in flow displacement between RL and RN fusions have recently been associated with often reported differences in patterns of aortopathy; RL is associated with dilation of the tubular portion of the

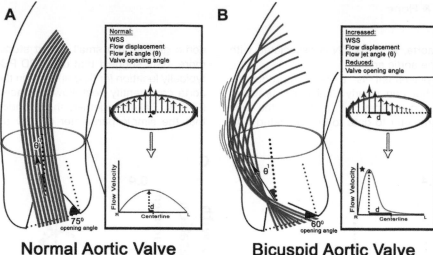

Fig. 2. Conventional aortic valve anatomy (*A*) is associated with a normal valve opening angle (~75°), flow jet angle (θ^1), wall shear stress (WSS), and flow displacement. Flow displacement measures the displacement of peak systolic flow (*arrowhead*) from the vessel centerline, and is normalized to aortic size. It is calculated by dividing the distance from centerline of peak systolic flow (*d*), by the aortic diameter (*dotted line with brackets*). The abnormal valve anatomy seen with a bicuspid aortic valve (*B*), here typical of right-left aortic leaflet fusion, leads to a reduced valve opening angle, increased flow jet angle (θ^1), and increased flow displacement. The increased near wall velocity gradient (*region denoted by star*) results in asymmetrically increased systolic WSS at the aortic convexity.

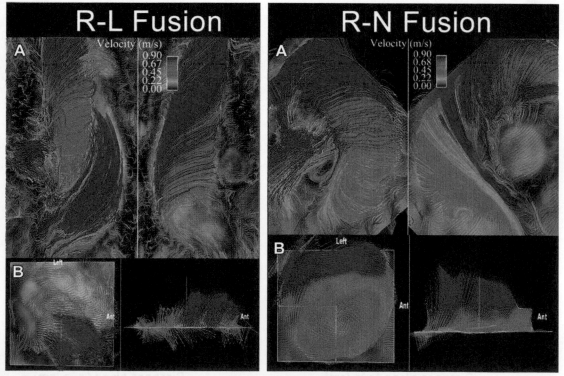

Fig. 3. Right-handed, nested helical flow in a patient with a bicuspid aortic valve involving fusion of the right and left leaflets (*R-L Fusion*), and normal aortic dimensions. (*A*) Streamline analysis reveals greater than 180° curvature of peak systolic streamlines in a right-handed twist around slower, central helical flow in the ascending thoracic aorta. (*B*) Vector analysis reveals a right-anterior eccentric systolic flow jet. Left-handed nested helical systolic flow in a patient with a bicuspid aortic valve involving fusion of the right and noncoronary leaflets (*R-N Fusion*) and normal aortic dimensions. (*A*) Streamline analysis reveals greater than 180° curvature of peak systolic streamlines in a left-handed twist around slower, central helical flow in the ascending thoracic aorta. (*B*) Vector analysis reveals a left-posterior eccentric flow jet. Ant, anterior. (*From* Hope MD, Hope TA, Meadows AK, et al. Bicuspid aortic valve: four-dimensional MR evaluation of ascending aortic systolic flow patterns. Radiology 2010;255(1):59, 60; with permission.)

ascending aorta, whereas RN is associated with dilation of the aortic arch.[32]

Flow displacement is a very reproducible parameter that can clearly distinguish between aortic valve phenotypes.[32,37] It is also the only 4D Flow parameter to date to be correlated with aortic growth in a small cohort study.[37] Furthermore, data suggest that using 2D PC-MRI at the typically location for flow analysis in the ascending aorta can identify peak flow displacement values (**Fig. 4**). Taken together, these findings suggest that the simple parameter of flow displacement

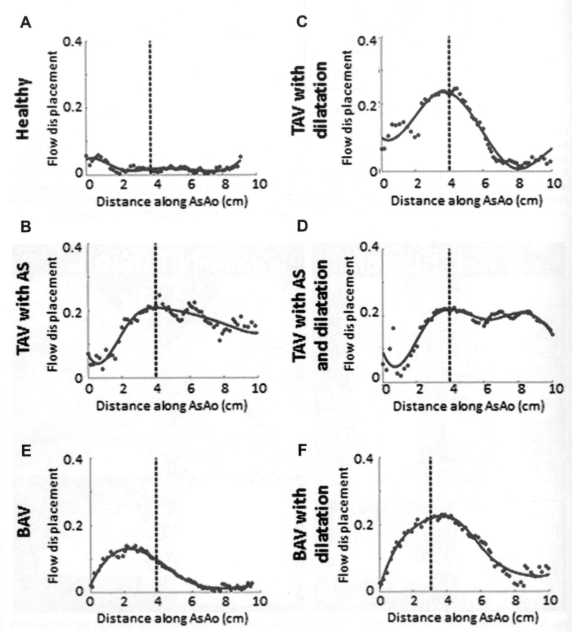

Fig. 4. Representative plots of flow displacement from each of the cross-sections (*red dots, red curve-spline fit*) as a function of distance along the ascending thoracic aorta (AsAo) for each of the 6 groups labeled. The *dotted blue line* indicates the location of the 2-dimensional plane, which was placed just distal to the sinotubular junction. No high-flow displacement was observed for the healthy control group (*A*). Generally, the presence of aortic stenosis resulted in the highest flow displacement values that remained high for longer distances along the AsAo (*B-D*). Patients with bicuspid aortic valves (BAV) had characteristic 3-dimensional displacement plots with a sharp increase to proximal high peak values, followed by a smooth tapering distally through the ascending aorta (*E, F*). TAV, tricuspid aortic valve. (*Courtesy of* M. Sigovan, PhD, University of Lyon, Lyon, France.)

could be calculated from conventional 2D PC-MRI for the risk stratification of patients with BAV for aortic disease progression.

Aortic Wall Disease

Diseases that stiffen the aortic wall can affect aortic flow. Aortic wall stiffening is commonly seen with aging and is an independent predictor of mortality both in the general population and for patients with common chronic illnesses.[38] Flow imaging can be used to estimate aortic wall stiffness by determining the speed of the systolic impulse through the aorta, or pulse wave velocity (PWV). Elevated PWV reflects wall stiffness and has been demonstrated using PC-MRI with hypertension and Marfan disease.[39,40] For Marfan patients, PWV has long been investigated as means of predicting disease progression, with normal PWV values associated with regional aortic stability.[41] 4D Flow offers a more comprehensive assessment

of aortic PWV than 2D PC-MRI (**Fig. 5**), and may improve the detection of regional differences that prior studies with Marfan syndrome have reported.[41,42] In addition to PWV, 4D Flow is capable of producing accurate, noninvasive measurements of aortic pressure waveforms.[43] Relative pressure can then be subdivided into inertial and viscous components, which show unique patterns in different types of aortopathy.[44]

Beside aortic wall stiffening, altered aortic flow patterns have been linked to the development of atherosclerosis. Low and oscillatory WSS have been shown induce endothelial changes that lead to plaque formation.[45,46] Using 4D Flow estimates of WSS, further evidence has been gathered showing the interrelationship of altered aortic flow and atherosclerotic plaque formation.[47,48] This suggests that 4D Flow could be used for identification of abnormal flow markers to predict an atherogenic-prone region, and thus guide risk stratification and medical management.

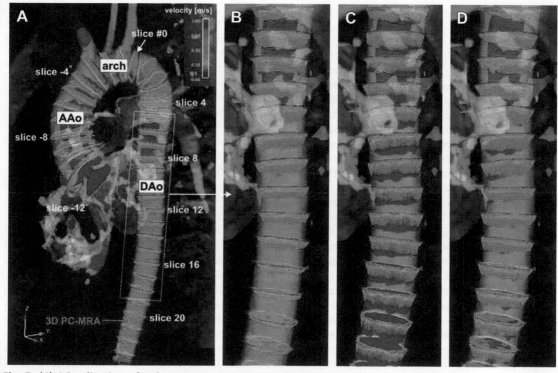

Fig. 5. (*A*): Visualization of pulse wave propagation within the thoracic aorta, based on flow-sensitive 3-directional phase contrast MRI (4D) data. Equidistant analysis planes with an interanalysis plane gap of 10 mm were positioned upstream (negative analysis plane numbers) and downstream (positive analysis plane numbers) along the thoracic aorta, starting with analysis plane #0 (outlet of the left subclavian artery). (*B–D*) Spatially varying flow profiles from the proximal to the descending thoracic aorta (DAo) in analysis planes can be appreciated in successive systolic time frames: during early systole (*B*), profiles in the proximal DAo are already fully developed, whereas velocities are continuously lower further downstream. During peak systole (*C*), flow profiles reach their maxima in the entire DAo, whereas during late systole (*D*), flow profiles in the proximal DAo are already reduced compared with flow further downstream. AAo, ascending thoracic aorta. (*From* Markl M, Wallis W, Brendecke S, et al. Estimation of global aortic pulse wave velocity by flow-sensitive 4D MRI. Magn Reson Med 2010;63(6):1579; with permission.)

SUMMARY

Aortic disease is routinely monitored with anatomic imaging, but until the recent advent of 4D Flow imaging, associated blood flow abnormalities have gone largely undetected. 4D Flow is a rapidly evolving technique that is currently able to measure a range of aortic hemodynamic markers in less than 15 minutes. Initial qualitative flow visualization has spurred the investigation of new quantitative flow markers. For example, eccentric systolic flow with BAV has led to the application of WSS and flow displacement for assessment of related ascending aortic disease. Many promising 4D Flow markers of aortic disease have been proposed, although larger prospective studies are needed to validate their clinical relevance. Within the next decade, 4D sequences may be commonly acquired during routine clinical cardiac MR studies, and provide valuable information to guide the medical and surgical management of patients with aortic disease.

REFERENCES

1. Olsson C, Thelin S, Stahle E, et al. Thoracic aortic aneurysm and dissection: increasing prevalence and improved outcomes reported in a nationwide population-based study of more than 14,000 cases from 1987 to 2002. Circulation 2006;114(24):2611–8.
2. Michelena HI, Khanna AD, Mahoney D, et al. Incidence of aortic complications in patients with bicuspid aortic valves. JAMA 2011;306(10):1104–12.
3. Clouse WD, Hallett JW Jr, Schaff HV, et al. Improved prognosis of thoracic aortic aneurysms: a population-based study. JAMA 1998;280(22):1926–9.
4. Tsai SF, Trivedi M, Daniels CJ. Comparing imaging modalities for screening aortic complications in patients with bicuspid aortic valve. Congenit Heart Dis 2012;7(4):372–7.
5. Bonow RO, Carabello BA, Chatterjee K, et al. ACC/AHA 2006 guidelines for the management of patients with valvular heart disease: a report of the American College of Cardiology/American Heart Association Task Force on Practice Guidelines (writing Committee to Revise the 1998 guidelines for the management of patients with valvular heart disease) developed in collaboration with the Society of Cardiovascular Anesthesiologists endorsed by the Society for Cardiovascular Angiography and Interventions and the Society of Thoracic Surgeons. J Am Coll Cardiol 2006;48(3):e1–148.
6. Steffens JC, Bourne MW, Sakuma H, et al. Quantification of collateral blood flow in coarctation of the aorta by velocity encoded cine magnetic resonance imaging. Circulation 1994;90(2):937–43.
7. Schnell S, Markl M, Entezari P, et al. k-t GRAPPA accelerated four-dimensional flow MRI in the aorta: effect on scan time, image quality, and quantification of flow and wall shear stress. Magn Reson Med 2014;72(2):522–33.
8. Hsiao A, Lustig M, Alley MT, et al. Rapid pediatric cardiac assessment of flow and ventricular volume with compressed sensing parallel imaging volumetric cine phase-contrast MRI. AJR Am J Roentgenol 2012;198(3):W250–9.
9. Gatehouse PD, Rolf MP, Graves MJ, et al. Flow measurement by cardiovascular magnetic resonance: a multi-centre multi-vendor study of background phase offset errors that can compromise the accuracy of derived regurgitant or shunt flow measurements. J Cardiovasc Magn Reson 2010;12:5.
10. Petersson S, Dyverfeldt P, Ebbers T. Assessment of the accuracy of MRI wall shear stress estimation using numerical simulations. J Magn Reson Imaging 2012;36(1):128–38.
11. Boussel L, Rayz V, Martin A, et al. Phase-contrast magnetic resonance imaging measurements in intracranial aneurysms in vivo of flow patterns, velocity fields, and wall shear stress: comparison with computational fluid dynamics. Magn Reson Med 2009;61(2):409–17.
12. Sengupta PP, Pedrizzetti G, Kilner PJ, et al. Emerging trends in CV flow visualization. JACC Cardiovasc Imaging 2012;5(3):305–16.
13. Hope MD, Wrenn SJ, Sigovan M, et al. Imaging Biomarkers of Aortic Disease: increased growth rates with eccentric systolic flow. J Am Coll Cardiol 2012;60(4):356–7.
14. Eriksson J, Carlhall CJ, Dyverfeldt P, et al. Semiautomatic quantification of 4D left ventricular blood flow. J Cardiovasc Magn Reson 2010;12:9.
15. Clough RE, Waltham M, Giese D, et al. A new imaging method for assessment of aortic dissection using four-dimensional phase contrast magnetic resonance imaging. J Vasc Surg 2012;55(4): 914–23.
16. Allen BD, Barker AJ, Kansal P, et al. Impact of aneurysm repair on thoracic aorta hemodynamics. Circulation 2013;128(17):e341–3.
17. Harloff A, Strecker C, Frydrychowicz AP, et al. Plaques in the descending aorta: a new risk factor for stroke? Visualization of potential embolization pathways by 4D MRI. J Magn Reson Imaging 2007 26(6):1651–5.
18. Chau KH, Elefteriades JA. Natural history of thoracic aortic aneurysms: size matters, plus moving beyond size. Prog Cardiovasc Dis 2013;56(1):74–80.
19. Verma S, Yanagawa B, Kalra S, et al. Knowledge attitudes, and practice patterns in surgical management of bicuspid aortopathy: a survey of 100 cardiac surgeons. J Thorac Cardiovasc Surg 2013 146(5):1033–40.e4.

20. Otto CM. Valvular aortic stenosis: disease severity and timing of intervention. J Am Coll Cardiol 2006; 47(11):2141–51.

21. Lancellotti P, Magne J. Valvuloarterial impedance in aortic stenosis: look at the load, but do not forget the flow. Eur J Echocardiogr 2011;12(5):354–7.

22. Briand M, Dumesnil JG, Kadem L, et al. Reduced systemic arterial compliance impacts significantly on left ventricular afterload and function in aortic stenosis: implications for diagnosis and treatment. J Am Coll Cardiol 2005;46(2):291–8.

23. Hachicha Z, Dumesnil JG, Pibarot P. Usefulness of the valvuloarterial impedance to predict adverse outcome in asymptomatic aortic stenosis. J Am Coll Cardiol 2009;54(11):1003–11.

24. Barker AJ, van Ooij P, Bandi K, et al. Viscous energy loss in the presence of abnormal aortic flow. Magn Reson Med 2014;72(3):620–8.

25. Dyverfeldt P, Hope M, Tseng EE, et al. Noninvasive magnetic resonance measurement of turbulent kinetic energy for the estimation of irreversible pressure loss in aortic stenosis. JACC Cardiovasc Imaging 2013;6(1):64–71.

26. Girdauskas E, Borger MA, Secknus MA, et al. Is aortopathy in bicuspid aortic valve disease a congenital defect or a result of abnormal hemodynamics? A critical reappraisal of a one-sided argument. Eur J Cardiothorac Surg 2011;39(6):809–14.

27. Lu MT, Thadani SR, Hope MD. Quantitative assessment of asymmetric aortic dilation with valve-related aortic disease. Acad Radiol 2013;20(1):10–5.

28. Della Corte A, Bancone C, Conti CA, et al. Restricted cusp motion in right-left type of bicuspid aortic valves: a new risk marker for aortopathy. J Thorac Cardiovasc Surg 2012;144(2):360–9.

29. Hope MD, Meadows AK, Hope TA, et al. Images in cardiovascular medicine. Evaluation of bicuspid aortic valve and aortic coarctation with 4D flow magnetic resonance imaging. Circulation 2008;117(21): 2818–9.

30. Bissell MM, Hess AT, Biasiolli L, et al. Aortic dilation in bicuspid aortic valve disease: flow pattern is a major contributor and differs with valve fusion type. Circ Cardiovasc Imaging 2013;6(4):499–507.

31. Hope MD, Hope TA, Meadows AK, et al. Bicuspid aortic valve: four-dimensional MR evaluation of ascending aortic systolic flow patterns. Radiology 2010;255(1):53–61.

32. Mahadevia R, Barker AJ, Schnell S, et al. Bicuspid aortic cusp fusion morphology alters aortic 3D outflow patterns, wall shear stress and expression of aortopathy. Circulation 2014;129(6):673–82.

33. Hope MD, Hope TA, Crook SE, et al. 4D flow CMR in assessment of valve-related ascending aortic disease. JACC Cardiovasc Imaging 2011;4(7):781–7.

34. Barker AJ, Markl M, Burk J, et al. Bicuspid aortic valve is associated with altered wall shear stress in the ascending aorta. Circ Cardiovasc Imaging 2012;5(4):457–66.

35. Stalder AF, Russe MF, Frydrychowicz A, et al. Quantitative 2D and 3D phase contrast MRI: optimized analysis of blood flow and vessel wall parameters. Magn Reson Med 2008;60(5):1218–31.

36. Sigovan M, Hope MD, Dyverfeldt P, et al. Comparison of four-dimensional flow parameters for quantification of flow eccentricity in the ascending aorta. J Magn Reson Imaging 2011;34(5):1226–30.

37. Hope MD, Sigovan M, Wrenn SJ, et al. MRI hemodynamic markers of progressive bicuspid aortic valve-related aortic disease. J Magn Reson Imaging 2014; 40(1):140–5.

38. Cavalcante JL, Lima JA, Redheuil A, et al. Aortic stiffness: current understanding and future directions. J Am Coll Cardiol 2011;57(14):1511–22.

39. Westenberg JJ, Scholte AJ, Vaskova Z, et al. Age-related and regional changes of aortic stiffness in the Marfan syndrome: assessment with velocity-encoded MRI. J Magn Reson Imaging 2011;34(3):526–31.

40. Brandts A, Westenberg JJ, van Elderen SG, et al. Site-specific coupling between vascular wall thickness and function: an observational MRI study of vessel wall thickening and stiffening in hypertension. Invest Radiol 2013;48(2):86–91.

41. Kroner ES, Scholte AJ, de Koning PJ, et al. MRI-assessed regional pulse wave velocity for predicting absence of regional aorta luminal growth in Marfan syndrome. Int J Cardiol 2013;167(6):2977–82.

42. Markl M, Wallis W, Brendecke S, et al. Estimation of global aortic pulse wave velocity by flow-sensitive 4D MRI. Magn Reson Med 2010;63(6):1575–82.

43. Delles M, Rengier F, Jeong YJ, et al. Estimation of aortic pressure waveforms from 4D phase-contrast MRI. Conf Proc IEEE Eng Med Biol Soc 2013;2013: 731–4.

44. Lamata P, Pitcher A, Krittian S, et al. Aortic relative pressure components derived from four-dimensional flow cardiovascular magnetic resonance. Magn Reson Med 2014;72(4):1162–9.

45. Cheng C, Tempel D, van Haperen R, et al. Atherosclerotic lesion size and vulnerability are determined by patterns of fluid shear stress. Circulation 2006; 113(23):2744–53.

46. Slager CJ, Wentzel JJ, Gijsen FJ, et al. The role of shear stress in the generation of rupture-prone vulnerable plaques. Nat Clin Pract Cardiovasc Med 2005;2(8):401–7.

47. Markl M, Brendecke SM, Simon J, et al. Co-registration of the distribution of wall shear stress and 140 complex plaques of the aorta. Magn Reson Imaging 2013;31(7):1156–62.

48. Frydrychowicz A, Stalder AF, Russe MF, et al. Three-dimensional analysis of segmental wall shear stress in the aorta by flow-sensitive four-dimensional-MRI. J Magn Reson Imaging 2009;30(1):77–84.

T1 Mapping
Technique and Applications

Juliano Lara Fernandes, MD, MBA, PhD[a], Carlos Eduardo Rochitte, MD, PhD[b],*

KEYWORDS

- Parametric mapping • T1 • Cardiovascular magnetic resonance • Fibrosis

KEY POINTS

- T1 mapping techniques have evolved along the years and become more simplified to be integrated into a clinical cardiovascular magnetic resonance examination.
- Native T1, postcontrast T1, and extracellular volume maps can be acquired and postprocessed manually or automatically in the scanner, simplifying the work flow.
- Longitudinal follow-up and comparison with normal values must be performed using the same T1 mapping method along with similar scanning parameters.

INTRODUCTION

Cardiovascular magnetic resonance (CMR) has evolved significantly in the last decade from a method restricted to anatomic imaging into a fully functional technique, incorporating in 1 single examination the possibility of looking at the many different facets of cardiovascular diseases with significant clinical impact.[1] Tissue characterization by CMR has been a key component in these many options afforded by the examination, one that is truly unique compared with other methods. However, until recently, this examination could be performed only in a qualitative or semiquantitative way, depending on the delimitation of user-selected thresholds and standard deviation curves, compared with supposedly normal tissue or in simple visual assessment.[2] This situation is especially the case when considering how late gadolinium enhancement (LGE) or edema imaging has been used; both techniques work well in regional lesions but fail to fully describe the more subtle involvement of the myocardium in diffuse disease.

T1 mapping, 1 form of tissue characterization performed with a parametric approach, has been gaining rapid popularity, as different sequences have been developed to integrate image acquisition into a clinical routine.[3] This technique allows fast progression from the basics of sequence development to its application in normal individuals and distinct diseases, sometimes overriding the more gradual steps taken with other CMR advances. In this review, state-of-the-art in T1 mapping is examined, focusing on its techniques, sequences, comparison of native versus extracellular volume (ECV) fraction measurements, as well as the current and future clinical applications of the method.

T1 SEQUENCES

T1 maps can be acquired using either inversion recovery (IR) or saturation recovery (SR) techniques.[4] Both methods use a first pulse to change the original longitudinal magnetization followed by acquisition of images along the relaxation curve and a fitting model to derive T1 values. **Table 1**

Disclosure statement: J.L. Fernandes has received speakers' honoraria from Novartis, participates in an Advisory Board for Sanofi-Aventis and has received research support from Siemens and Novartis.
[a] Cardiovascular Imaging Center, Jose Michel Kalaf Research Institute, Av Jose de Souza Campo 840, Campinas, Sao Paulo 13025260, Brazil; [b] CMR and CCT Section, Cardiology Department, Heart Institute (InCor), University of Sao Paulo Medical School, Av Dr Eneas de Carvalho Aguiar 44–Andar AB, São Paulo, Sao Paulo 05403-900, Brazil
* Corresponding author.
E-mail address: rochitte@incor.usp.br

Table 1
Different T1 mapping sequences

Sequence	Type	Number of Heartbeats	Advantages	Disadvantages
MOLLI (original)	IR	17: 3 (3)3 (3)5	First MOLLI sequence developed	Heart rate dependence Long acquisition times Underestimation of true T1 value (especially at fast heart rates)
MOLLI (native T1)	IR	8: 5 (3)3	No heart rate dependency Fast acquisition	Underestimation of true T1 because of magnetization transfer effects
MOLLI (postcontrast)	IR	9: 4 (1s)3 (1s)2	No heart rate dependency Fast acquisition Less recovery phase needed with short T1	Few validation studies
MOLLI (T1*)	IR	Any of the above without need for correction	Used for LV blood assessment, with new inflow blood (eg, for ECV calculation)	
shMOLLI	IR	5: (1)1 (1)1	No heart rate dependency Accurate in both precontrast and postcontrast situations	Less signal-to-noise ratio compared with MOLLI More prone to artifacts Systematic underestimation of true T1 for values >800 ms (corrected by formula)
SASHA	SR	10	No T1* effect No heart rate dependence No T2 sensitivity in 3-parameter fit Less sensitive to off-resonance effects	Less signal-to-noise ratio compared with IR sequences Less precision if used in a 2-parameter fit model

summarizes current T1 map techniques and their advantages/disadvantages.

Look and Locker[5] developed the first IR sequences, which were applied clinically many years ago, but this technique has limited use in the heart and does not allow pixelwise fitting, because it requires continuous acquisition throughout the cardiac cycle. An advancement of this method to incorporate a segmented approach with a fixed acquisition period evolved into a modified Look-Locker IR (MOLLI) scheme.[6] In MOLLI, multiple inversion times (TIs) are used with different trigger delays. These inversion pulses are interleaved with recovery periods to establish a more homogeneous initial magnetization along different heartbeats. The original MOLLI sequence used 17 heartbeats with acquisition of 3-3-5 images, with 3 heartbeats for recovery between each experiment: 3 (3)3 (3)5 notation. This first method suffered from a few problems, which were dealt with in subsequent developments of the initial principles. First, in some patients, the acquisition

times could still take a long period of breath holding, resulting in subpar results. Second, because the readout for MOLLI uses a steady state free precession technique, it underestimates the final T1 value (generating in effect a T1* time), with need for a correction factor. Third, the fitting parameters were also dependent on heart rate (consequently on the inversion/recovery periods) and could vary significantly, especially in situations of extreme T1 values.

To correct for these factors, new mixes in inversion/recovery times and number of heartbeats of the original sequences were proposed: for precontrast (native) acquisitions, a 5 (3)3 model has been proposed, with only 8 heartbeats and less dependence on the heart rate[7]; for postcontrast acquisitions, a 4 (1s)3 (1s)2 format may be used, because the recovery time can be shortened to only 1 second, as noted.[8] For the blood pool, in which new fresh blood is entering the image plane, it is recommended that the original images be used without the correction factor (actual T1* images).

Another approach to the IR method using a faster acquisition protocol is shortened MOLLI (shMOLLI).[9] This sequence requires only 9 heartbeats using a 5 (1)1 (1)1 scheme, with conditional fitting of the last 2 images after relatively short TIs, depending on the length of the T1 (shorter T1s use all samples; longer T1s use only the first 5 images). This situation results not only in shorter overall acquisitions but also in less dependency on heart rate and on precontrast and postcontrast situations with wide ranges of T1 times. In exchange for these advantages, the shMOLLI sequence is known to underestimate the true T1 times by 4% when this value is more than 800 milliseconds, as well as presenting less signal-to-noise ratio (SNR) compared with the original MOLLI scheme.

Apart from the first IR sequences, SR alternatives have been proposed in the light of their increased accuracy in exchange for shorter range of T1 values measured. The first technique to be applied clinically is saturation recovery single shot acquisition (SASHA), which acquires 1 image before any saturation followed by multiple SR pulses with different trigger delay times.[10] There is no dependency on the readout for SASHA, so larger flip angles can be used, although this necessitates the fitting parameters to be altered, with a loss of precision. Moreover, because the SNR in these sequences is reduced compared with the IR sequences, there is an additional loss in precision with more artifacts. Because of its less widespread use in different clinical scenarios compared with MOLLI techniques, this technique might need more clinical validation studies but certainly holds promise as an alternative method for T1 mapping.

Two recently published techniques might also add options to the T1 map sequence menu. The first one is a combined SR/IR sequence called saturation pulse prepared heart rate independent inversion recovery, which, as the name implies, is not sensitive to variations in rate at the expense of slightly longer acquisition times.[11] The second is a new SR technique in which each RR interval receives a saturation pulse with the acquisition of longer delay times in the recovery curve performed across multiple heart beats (SMART$_1$Map).[12] This technique obviates T1* correction as in MOLLI and makes the sequence less sensitive to other imaging parameters.

Two additional points are worth mentioning when discussing T1 mapping techniques. First, in principle, motion correction can be applied to all sequences described earlier, which should help with the creation of automatic pixel-fitted color maps. Second, many factors still influence the T1 results, and even small changes in parameters might hinder

the possibility of T1 comparison among different time points or individuals. Therefore, it is essential in longitudinal studies to stick to the same original sequence used instead of changing many parameters or type of sequence designs.

NATIVE, POSTCONTRAST, AND EXTRACELLULAR VOLUME FRACTION MAPS

When performing T1 mapping, there are many choices for how to evaluate the myocardium with the previously described sequences. The simplest form is by running the sequences without any contrast and obtaining the native T1 measures (also previously called precontrast or noncontrast).[13] Many investigators have described the use of native T1 in different clinical scenarios, as explained later; this setting is particularly useful in patients with renal disease, for example.

Another way to apply T1 mapping is through the injection of gadolinium-base contrast media at doses that vary from 0.15 to 0.2 mmol/kg, with subsequent imaging of the myocardium after at least 15 minutes from the bolus injection.[14] This approach seems to offer similar results compared with the alternative equilibrium contrast infusion and is more easily applicable in daily practice.[15] Both techniques allow for the quantification of postcontrast T1 values in comparable ways.

Although both native and postcontrast T1 measurements show promising clinical applications, by measuring both values along with the T1 figures for the blood pool and the patient's hematocrit (Ht) level, the ECV of the myocardium can then be calculated, which is more stable over time and may have more relevance in clinical practice.[16,17] ECV can be automatically calculated inline by the scanner, but this usually needs to be performed manually during postprocessing: the partition coefficient λ is calculated from (1/T1 pre Gd − 1/T1 post Gd)$_{myocardium}$/(1/T1 pre Gd − 1/T1 post Gd)$_{blood}$, where Gd is gadolinium; the ECV is then calculated as λ (1-Ht).

CLINICAL APPLICATIONS OF T1 MAPPING

The normal myocardial structure contains both myocytes and connective tissue, with cardiac myocytes representing most of the myocardial mass. Therefore, intracellular space corresponds to most of the myocardial volume. Cardiomyopathies, despite their multiple causes and complex processes causing the myocardial injury, have a usual final pathway that involves myocardial fibrosis deposition and increase in extracellular space. Myocardial fibrosis can be classified in several subtypes, such as reactive interstitial fibrosis, infiltrative interstitial fibrosis, and replacement or scarring fibrosis.[18] These processes can cause a change in the ratio of myocytes to interstitial volume, may occur diffusely on the myocardium, and may be an early abnormality in some cases. As we previously commented, this diffuse change on the extracellular space is missed by techniques depending on regional heterogeneity of myocardial abnormalities, such as LGE, and can be detected only by measurements of myocardium longitudinal relaxation time before and after contrast and estimation of myocardium ECV.

Several cardiomyopathies have been investigated in the recent literature, with a variety of different T1 mapping techniques. Despite the lack of standard measurements, the available data have repeatedly shown that changes in the T1 and ECV are present in the diseased myocardium and might have clinical and prognostic significance. Most of these data are reviewed in the following section.

AORTIC VALVE DISEASE

Myocardial fibrosis detectable by LGE has been reported in patients with severe aortic valve disease.[19–21] The presence and magnitude of myocardial fibrosis correlated with clinical prognosis after aortic valve replacement. Moreover, the presence of myocardial fibrosis by LGE correlated with the burden of interstitial myocardial fibrosis measured by pathology on myocardium samples obtained during aortic valve replacement surgery.[21] This finding might suggest that measurements of interstitial diffuse fibrosis would add significant clinical information. In 2006, a pilot study reported shorter T1s in 8 patients with aortic regurgitation compared with controls. In a more recent technical validation study, patients with severe aortic stenosis showed moderate correlation between ECV calculated by 2 T1 mapping sequences before and after contrast and collagen volume fraction derived from myocardial biopsy samples.[22] The ability to obtain myocardial biopsies during aortic valve replacement surgery also provided further histologic validation of ECV in patients with severe aortic stenosis.[23] In contrast, native T1 in patients with aortic stenosis were not different from normal controls.[24] In a larger study, ECV in 66 patients with severe aortic stenosis correlated with end-systolic volume index and aortic valve area measured by echocardiography. Only 42% of these patients had some degree of LGE in the left ventricular (LV) myocardium.[25] Optimization of the T1 techniques in 3 T are still being investigated, using patients with aortic stenosis as the validation group.[26]

T1 mapping and ECV are altered in patients with severe aortic stenosis and correlate to LGE presence and a variety of clinical and imaging parameters of disease severity. Techniques are not standardized; there are no histologic validation data other than in severe aortic stenosis with indication to surgery, such as mild, moderate, or severe and asymptomatic patients; scarce data available on aortic regurgitation; and barely any data on clinical significance or prognosis of ECV in patients with aortic valve disease. Although these data are promising, additional clinical data are needed to bring T1 mapping and ECV calculation to clinical use.

HYPERTROPHIC CARDIOMYOPATHY

Myocardial fibrosis has been shown to be an important feature of hypertrophic cardiomyopathy (HCM), which can differentiate this disease from other causes of myocardial hypertrophy in pathology. Although fibrosis is not specific to HCM, its quantification and regional distribution provide useful information in the pathophysiology.[27] Recent CMR studies have shown that myocardial fibrosis in patients with HCM correlate with disease severity and prognosis.[28,29] However, approximately 65% of patients with HCM have any degree of LGE[30] and, therefore, a threshold for myocardial fibrosis that indicates worse prognosis and that implantable cardioverter-defibrillator (ICD) implantation is still needed. Recently, an initial attempt of validation was performed using myocardial delayed enhancement by multidetector computed tomography, resulting in a cutoff of 18 g or 14% of LV mass for higher rates of appropriate therapy by ICD in patients with HCM.[31] In a recent personal communication of data (Martin Maron, 2014) on a multicenter prospective trial using LGE by magnetic resonance imaging in patients with HCM, Dr Martin Maron reported that an LGE cutoff of 15% of LV mass indicates a worse prognosis in HCM. Therefore, the myocardial fibrosis process is critical in HCM and has established clinical and prognostic significance.

Investigation of T1 values on HCM is still in its infancy. Native T1 values are higher in patients with HCM compared with controls, even in LV segments without LGE, but not different from patients with dilated cardiomyopathy (DCM).[32] Although the differences in T1 values were small, T1 values provided an index with high diagnostic accuracy for the detection of diffusely diseased myocardium.[33]

Initial data in 2009 using T1 scout (Look-Locker) sequences in patients with HCM suggested that 10-minute postcontrast T1 values could identify dispersed myocardial damage.[34] A technique of equilibrium contrast was first tested and validated in patients with HCM and was able to measure diffuse myocardial fibrosis,[15] using multiple breath-hold acquisition of standard LGE with different TIs and also using single breath-hold shMOLLI for the calculation of ECV.[22] The equilibrium technique in HCM was shown to be comparable with bolus only technique for a wide range of T1 values and ECV. The calculation of ECV in patients with HCM showed that the area of ECV greater than a fix threshold of 30.4% was consistently larger than the area of LGE measured as greater than 2 standard deviations of the remote nonenhanced myocardium.[17] In patients with HCM, ECV did not correlate to any other CMR parameters (LV ejection fraction [LVEF] and volume indexes), except moderately with the percentage of LGE ($r = 0.48$), but were larger than in normal individuals (0.291 ± 0.005 vs 0.250 ± 0.023, $P<.001$).[25] This finding may be helpful in differentiating patients with HCM from those with other diseases that are usually confounded using regular techniques, such as athlete's heart (**Fig. 1**). This observation is especially true because the heterogeneity of scar and its diffuse distribution in patients with HCM makes definition of normal myocardium challenging in this disease and, thus, hampers the measurements of myocardial fibrosis based on LGE and standard deviation thresholds over the normal myocardial. In this scenario, T1 maps and, particularly ECV are a more attractive option and potentially more accurate for estimating disease severity. Yet, the clinical and prognostic value of T1 mapping and ECV calculation over the standard LGE still needs to be shown.

ANDERSON-FABRY DISEASE

An important clinical scenario is the differential diagnosis of Anderson-Fabry disease (AFD) and other LV hypertrophy (LVH) causes, including HCM. A more concentric LVH with predominant lateral wall fibrosis in middle-aged men should indicate the need to rule out AFD. CMR with standard LGE was histologically validated[35] in AFD and is useful in the diagnosis and early therapy initiation[36] and response prediction.[37]

Native T1 values and mapping have a unique ability to differentiate AFD from other causes of LVH. Lower T1 values in the mid and basal septum of patients with AFD was shown in a recent study comparing AFD, healthy volunteers, and other patients (hypertension, HCM, aortic stenosis): 882 ± 47, 968 ± 32 and 1018 ± 74 milliseconds, respectively ($P<.0001$).[38] This finding can be explained because fat has very low T1 relaxation time, and AFD pathophysiology involves the intracellular storage of glycosphingolipid in the myocardium. In that study,[38] a value of 940 milliseconds differentiated AFD, with no overlap, from other diseases.

On the other hand, ECV measurements in AFD showed no difference from the normal volunteers (0.250 ± 0.023 vs 0.253 ± 0.035, respectively, not significant) in a study from the same group of researchers. In addition, the ECV in AFD showed no correlation to other CMR parameters, such as LVEF, volume indexes, LV mass, and left atrium size. Although the initial lipid storage is intracellular and could explain the lack of difference on ECV, during the disease progression, myocardial fibrosis develops, particularly on the LV lateral wall, which should increase ECV. Sado and colleagues[39] measured ECV only on the mid and

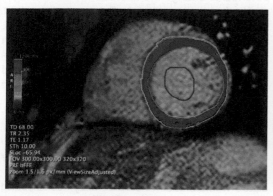
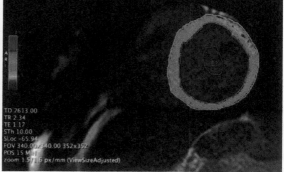

Native T1 **Post Contrast**

Fig. 1. Example of an ECV calculation on a patient referred for the differential diagnosis of athlete's heart versus HCM. The native T1 of 1071 milliseconds is shown on the left, with measurement of all the myocardium at mid-level. A 15-minute postcontrast image is shown on the right, with a decrease in the original T1 values to 523 milliseconds. The measurement of the blood pool T1 as well as the Ht allowed for the calculation of an ECV 26.7%, which is less than the usual cutoff for HCM.

basal septum, where AFD has shown little myocardial fibrosis, as shown by pathology.

Therefore, although ECV data on AFD are still missing and its clinical importance needs to be further investigated, native T1 holds enormous potential for clinical use and management of patients with AFD.

DILATED CARDIOMYOPATHY

Since the classic description of the midwall linear septal fibrosis in dilated cardiomyopathy (DCM),[40] standard LGE has been shown to have consistently prognostic significance in patients with DCM.[41,42]

Dass and colleagues[32] reported recently that native T1 mapping detects the underlying disease process in DCM beyond LGE in low-risk individuals. DCM T1 values were not significantly higher than in patients with HCM, but higher than in normal volunteers. Nonetheless, segments without LGE had higher T1 values than segments in normal control individuals. Recently, Puntmann and colleagues[33] also showed that nonischemic DCM presented T1 values higher than normal volunteers and similar to patients with HCM.

Postcontrast T1 measurements were first investigated in 20 patients with DCM in 2009 and showed a reduced blood-myocardium δ TI and T1, providing first evidence for the presence of diffuse fibrosis.[43] ECV was subsequently investigated in patients with DCM showing increased values compared with normal controls (40% vs 27%[33] and 38% vs 25%[17]).

As for previous diseases, native T1, T1 mapping, and ECV have strong potential to enhance our understanding of the disease processes, but several questions remain and should be addressed in further studies, particularly on their clinical relevance for patient management and prognostication.

AMYLOIDOSIS

Cardiac amyloidosis (CA) is hallmark disease for diffuse increased extracellular space of the myocardium and is the leading cause of morbidity and mortality in systemic amyloidosis. LGE has been described in this disease, and the challenging adjustment of TI is part of this description, along with global subendocardial enhancement on standard LGE images.[44,45] More recently, different patterns of LGE have been able to differentiate amyloid light-chain (AL) and transthyretin-related amyloidosis (ATTR CA), with clear clinical implications for patient management.[46] Despite the ominous prognosis of CA, the presence and pattern of LGE were associated with markers of prognosis.

Native T1 has high diagnostic accuracy for detecting cardiac AL amyloidosis, with higher sensitivity than standard LGE imaging. Native T1 mapping was able to differentiate patients with amyloidosis, but otherwise no cardiac involvement from normal individuals, and also from those with possible and definitive cardiac involvement.[24] In patients with LVH, CA showed the highest T1 values compared with hypertension, HCM, and aortic stenosis.[38]

ECV measurements in CA were initially described using the equilibrium contrast technique and had close values for multi–breath-hold and single breath-hold techniques (48 ± 6 and 52 ± 7%, respectively). Another study showed ECV values ranging from 41% to 49% for patients with biopsied proven CA and clinical CA, respectively.[47] Sado and colleagues[25] reported that ECV in CA correlated with other CMR parameters: LVEF (r = −0.57), ESV index (r = −0.63), LV mass (r = −0.44) and septal thickness (r = −0.51). In CA, which in general has the highest ECV, the equilibrium versus bolus techniques showed the greatest differences, with bolus technique tending to overestimate ECVs more than 40%.[23] In a larger cohort, White and colleagues[48] reported that the use of standard LGE with different TIs and the simple and rapid visual inspection of the image sequence allowed for the distinction of histologically proven CA LVH from LVH of other causes, and this finding was a strong predictor of mortality. The visual inspection of LGE images with sequential TIs in CA shows the null point of the myocardium before the blood null point, opposite to the other LVH causes.

Techniques assessing the ECV in CA have great potential to change the approach to the management of patients with CA. Future studies of T1 mapping and ECV protocols using larger cohorts, which include other gammopathies and which investigate imaging characteristics of clinical outcomes, are needed. In addition, for a full clinical application, quantitative CMR techniques must be standardized and simplified.

MYOCARDITIS

Myocardial fibrosis detected by LGE is crucial for the differential diagnosis of acute chest pain associated with increase in cardiac enzymes in young adults, in conjunction with other myocardial edema sequences and others in a complete CMR examination.[49] Histologic validation,[50] clinical diagnostic significance,[51] and prognostic value[52] place LGE by CMR centrally in the algorithm for management of acute myocarditis.[53]

In a recent study, Ferreira and colleagues[54] evaluated 50 patients with acute myocarditis and native T1 mapping. T1 mapping showed excellent and superior diagnostic performance compared with T2-weighted images, with higher sensitivity than T2-weighted images and LGE. This technique can be useful for detecting focal subtle disease and also global and diffuse changes, which are a challenge for techniques dependent on regional myocardial comparisons versus normal myocardium. The same research group previously investigated in Takotsubo cardiomyopathy the global myocardial edema using native T1 mapping and reported high diagnostic performance, suggesting at least a complementary role over the T2-weighted images for assessing myocardial edema.

In a recent case report, Schumm and colleagues[55] first reported the capabilities of the promising new technique of T1 mapping in the setting of acute onset of biopsy-proven viral myocarditis. Against the background of the recent controversy over T2-weighted images, in which the argument has been made that there is no proven physiologic basis for most apparent T2 findings,[56] quantitative T1 mapping, being also sensitive to changes in water content and acquired without the use of gadolinium contrast, may overcome the limitations of T2-weighted CMR and may be a more accurate technique for detection of tissue edema or hyperemia in areas with and without irreversible myocardial injury.[54] T1 mapping could improve the decision-making process for referring patients for endomyocardial biopsy and add information on disease progression, LV remodeling, and outcome.

Future larger cohort studies are warranted to show the clinical values, prognostic significance, and usefulness on patient management. Until then, T1 mapping remains in the realm of research for acute myocarditis evaluation.

MYOCARDIAL INFARCTION

Since the first description of alterations in magnetic relaxation times in acute myocardial infarction (MI) in dogs by Higgins and colleagues,[57] LGE CMR technique has become the gold standard method for MI detection[58] and viability assessment.[59]

The seminal study describing the MOLLI sequence included an infarcted patient for its validation.[6] The same investigators subsequently studied 24 patients 8 days and 6 months after their first MI. T1 mapping was performed at baseline and 2 to 20 minutes after gadolinium-based contrast administration. Several conclusions emerged from this pioneer study: T1 map matches LGE infarct size better in chronic MIs than in acute MIs; acute and chronic infarcts present different T1 changes; and precontrast T1 maps enable the detection of acute MI.[60] MI healing was also investigated, and T1 mapping using standard LGE at several TI times showed that within a week after acute MI, the remote region undergoes expansion of the extracellular matrix, associated with systolic dysfunction.[61]

Measurements of ECV in chronic MI reached 68.5% ± 8.6%, without associated microvascular obstruction.[17] In patients with a week of acute MI, ECV measurements within the infarcted area using the equilibrium contrast technique were 58.5% ± 7.6%, higher than in patients with CA.[25] ECV was also investigated in the scenario of subtle and atypical LGE compared with patients with MI, and results showed that ECV was able to differentiate MI (ECV = 51% ± 8%) from normal remote myocardium (ECV = 27% ± 3%). In nonischemic cardiomyopathy, the atypical LGE (ECV = 37% ± 6%) showed clear differences from normal appearing myocardium (ECV = 26% ± 3%), which increased with age and decreased LVEF in patients with previous MI.[16] This finding is consistent with diffuse fibrosis related to aging and LV remodeling/infarct healing after MI. One important proof that subtle increases in ECV relates to extracellular matrix expansion and to subclinical myocardial disease is the work of Wong and colleagues,[62] which evaluated 793 consecutive patients without amyloidosis or HCM and showed that in volunteers, ECV ranged from 21.7% to 26.2%, whereas for patients, it ranged from 21.0% to 45.8%. Moreover, ECV was independently related to all-cause mortality and major events.

Although LGE will remain as the main stem clinical application for chronic and acute MIs, T1 mapping and ECV have the potential to further evaluate remote and peri-infarct zone with distinct lens and provide additional pathophysiologic understanding of infarction processes and healing.

FUTURE DIRECTIONS

For T1 mapping to enter mainstream use and become a truly routine sequence incorporated into daily clinical CMR use, there are still some goals to accomplish. Although many sequences are available, rapid evolution with significant enhancement in parameters makes longitudinal studies difficult to follow and comparison among different centers tricky. New studies that use this parameter as a meaningful end point also need to be created if T1 values are to be used as an important imaging marker in clinical decision making. Nevertheless, progress has been rapid, and different stakeholders have been working together to reach this same objective, so there is a long but promising path to follow.[63]

REFERENCES

1. Bruder O, Wagner A, Lombardi M, et al. European Cardiovascular Magnetic Resonance (EuroCMR) registry–multi national results from 57 centers in 15 countries. J Cardiovasc Magn Reson 2013;15:9.
2. Turkbey EB, Nacif MS, Noureldin RA, et al. Differentiation of myocardial scar from potential pitfalls and artefacts in delayed enhancement MRI. Br J Radiol 2012;85(1019):e1145–54.
3. Salerno M, Kramer CM. Advances in parametric mapping with CMR imaging. JACC Cardiovasc Imaging 2013;6(7):806–22.
4. Kellman P, Hansen MS. T1-mapping in the heart: accuracy and precision. J Cardiovasc Magn Reson 2014;16(1):2.
5. Look D, Locker D. Time saving in measurement of NMR and EPR relaxation times. Rev Sci Instrum 1970;41:250–1.
6. Messroghli DR, Radjenovic A, Kozerke S, et al. Modified Look-Locker inversion recovery (MOLLI) for high-resolution T1 mapping of the heart. Magn Reson Med 2004;52(1):141–6.
7. Kellman P, Wilson JR, Xue H, et al. Extracellular volume fraction mapping in the myocardium, part 1: evaluation of an automated method. J Cardiovasc Magn Reson 2012;14:63.
8. Kellman P, Arai AE, Xue H. T1 and extracellular volume mapping in the heart: estimation of error maps and the influence of noise on precision. J Cardiovasc Magn Reson 2013;15:56.
9. Piechnik SK, Ferreira VM, Dall'Armellina E, et al. Shortened modified Look-Locker inversion recovery (ShMOLLI) for clinical myocardial T1-mapping at 1.5 and 3 T within a 9 heartbeat breathhold. J Cardiovasc Magn Reson 2010;12:69.
10. Chow K, Flewitt JA, Green JD, et al. Saturation recovery single-shot acquisition (SASHA) for myocardial T mapping. Magn Reson Med 2013;71(6): 2082–95.
11. Weingartner S, Akcakaya M, Basha T, et al. Combined saturation/inversion recovery sequences for improved evaluation of scar and diffuse fibrosis in patients with arrhythmia or heart rate variability. Magn Reson Med 2014;71(3):1024–34.
12. Slavin GS, Stainsby JA. True T1 mapping with SMART1Map (saturation method using adaptive recovery times for cardiac T1 mapping): a comparison with MOLLI. J Cardiovasc Magn Reson 2013; 15(Suppl 1):P3.
13. Moon JC, Messroghli DR, Kellman P, et al. Myocardial T1 mapping and extracellular volume quantification: a Society for Cardiovascular Magnetic Resonance (SCMR) and CMR Working Group of the European Society of Cardiology consensus statement. J Cardiovasc Magn Reson 2013;15:92.
14. Schelbert EB, Testa SM, Meier CG, et al. Myocardial extravascular extracellular volume fraction measurement by gadolinium cardiovascular magnetic resonance in humans: slow infusion versus bolus. J Cardiovasc Magn Reson 2011;13:16.
15. Flett AS, Hayward MP, Ashworth MT, et al. Equilibrium contrast cardiovascular magnetic resonance for the measurement of diffuse myocardial fibrosis: preliminary validation in humans. Circulation 2010; 122(2):138–44.
16. Ugander M, Oki AJ, Hsu LY, et al. Extracellular volume imaging by magnetic resonance imaging provides insights into overt and sub-clinical myocardial pathology. Eur Heart J 2012;33(10):1268–78.
17. Kellman P, Wilson JR, Xue H, et al. Extracellular volume fraction mapping in the myocardium, part 2: initial clinical experience. J Cardiovasc Magn Reson 2012;14:64.
18. Mewton N, Liu CY, Croisille P, et al. Assessment of myocardial fibrosis with cardiovascular magnetic resonance. J Am Coll Cardiol 2011;57(8):891–903.
19. Nigri M, Azevedo CF, Rochitte CE, et al. Contrast-enhanced magnetic resonance imaging identifies focal regions of intramyocardial fibrosis in patients with severe aortic valve disease: correlation with quantitative histopathology. Am Heart J 2009; 157(2):361–8.
20. Weidemann F, Herrmann S, Stork S, et al. Impact of myocardial fibrosis in patients with symptomatic severe aortic stenosis. Circulation 2009;120(7): 577–84.
21. Azevedo CF, Nigri M, Higuchi ML, et al. Prognostic significance of myocardial fibrosis quantification by histopathology and magnetic resonance imaging in patients with severe aortic valve disease. J Am Coll Cardiol 2010;56(4):278–87.
22. Fontana M, White SK, Banypersad SM, et al. Comparison of T1 mapping techniques for ECV quantification. Histological validation and reproducibility of ShMOLLI versus multibreath-hold T1 quantification equilibrium contrast CMR. J Cardiovasc Magn Reson 2012;14:88.
23. White SK, Sado DM, Fontana M, et al. T1 mapping for myocardial extracellular volume measurement by CMR: bolus only versus primed infusion technique. JACC Cardiovasc Imaging 2013;6(9):955–62.
24. Karamitsos TD, Piechnik SK, Banypersad SM, et al. Noncontrast T1 mapping for the diagnosis of cardiac amyloidosis. JACC Cardiovasc Imaging 2013;6(4):488–97.
25. Sado DM, Flett AS, Banypersad SM, et al. Cardiovascular magnetic resonance measurement of myocardial extracellular volume in health and disease. Heart 2012;98(19):1436–41.

26. Chin CW, Semple S, Malley T, et al. Optimization and comparison of myocardial T1 techniques at 3T in patients with aortic stenosis. Eur Heart J Cardiovasc Imaging 2014;15(5):556–65.

27. Tanaka M, Fujiwara H, Onodera T, et al. Quantitative analysis of myocardial fibrosis in normals, hypertensive hearts, and hypertrophic cardiomyopathy. Heart 1986;55(6):575–81.

28. Bruder O, Wagner A, Jensen CJ, et al. Myocardial scar visualized by cardiovascular magnetic resonance imaging predicts major adverse events in patients with hypertrophic cardiomyopathy. J Am Coll Cardiol 2010;56(11):875–87.

29. O'Hanlon R, Grasso A, Roughton M, et al. Prognostic significance of myocardial fibrosis in hypertrophic cardiomyopathy. J Am Coll Cardiol 2010; 56(11):867–74.

30. Noureldin RA, Liu S, Nacif MS, et al. The diagnosis of hypertrophic cardiomyopathy by cardiovascular magnetic resonance. J Cardiovasc Magn Reson 2012;14:17.

31. Shiozaki AA, Senra T, Arteaga E, et al. Myocardial fibrosis detected by cardiac CT predicts ventricular fibrillation/ventricular tachycardia events in patients with hypertrophic cardiomyopathy. J Cardiovasc Comput Tomogr 2013;7(3): 173–81.

32. Dass S, Suttie JJ, Piechnik SK, et al. Myocardial tissue characterization using magnetic resonance noncontrast T1 mapping in hypertrophic and dilated cardiomyopathy. Circ Cardiovasc Imaging 2012;5(6):726–33.

33. Puntmann VO, Voigt T, Chen Z, et al. Native T1 mapping in differentiation of normal myocardium from diffuse disease in hypertrophic and dilated cardiomyopathy. JACC Cardiovasc Imaging 2013; 6(4):475–84.

34. Amano Y, Takayama M, Kumita S. Contrast-enhanced myocardial T1-weighted scout (Look-Locker) imaging for the detection of myocardial damages in hypertrophic cardiomyopathy. J Magn Reson Imaging 2009;30(4):778–84.

35. Moon JC, Sheppard M, Reed E, et al. The histological basis of late gadolinium enhancement cardiovascular magnetic resonance in a patient with Anderson-Fabry disease. J Cardiovasc Magn Reson 2006;8(3):479–82.

36. Moon JC, Sachdev B, Elkington AG, et al. Gadolinium enhanced cardiovascular magnetic resonance in Anderson-Fabry disease. Evidence for a disease specific abnormality of the myocardial interstitium. Eur Heart J 2003;24(23):2151–5.

37. Beer M, Weidemann F, Breunig F, et al. Impact of enzyme replacement therapy on cardiac morphology and function and late enhancement in Fabry's cardiomyopathy. Am J Cardiol 2006; 97(10):1515–8.

38. Sado DM, White SK, Piechnik SK, et al. Identification and assessment of Anderson-Fabry disease by cardiovascular magnetic resonance noncontrast myocardial T1 mapping. Circ Cardiovasc Imaging 2013;6(3):392–8.

39. Sheppard MN, Cane P, Florio R, et al. A detailed pathologic examination of heart tissue from three older patients with Anderson-Fabry disease on enzyme replacement therapy. Cardiovasc Pathol 2010;19(5):293–301.

40. McCrohon JA, Moon JC, Prasad SK, et al. Differentiation of heart failure related to dilated cardiomyopathy and coronary artery disease using gadolinium-enhanced cardiovascular magnetic resonance. Circulation 2003;108(1):54–9.

41. Assomull RG, Prasad SK, Lyne J, et al. Cardiovascular magnetic resonance, fibrosis, and prognosis in dilated cardiomyopathy. J Am Coll Cardiol 2006; 48(10):1977–85.

42. Wu KC, Weiss RG, Thiemann DR, et al. Late gadolinium enhancement by cardiovascular magnetic resonance heralds an adverse prognosis in nonischemic cardiomyopathy. J Am Coll Cardiol 2008; 51(25):2414–21.

43. Han Y, Peters DC, Dokhan B, et al. Shorter difference between myocardium and blood optimal inversion time suggests diffuse fibrosis in dilated cardiomyopathy. J Magn Reson Imaging 2009; 30(5):967–72.

44. Vogelsberg H, Mahrholdt H, Deluigi CC, et al. Cardiovascular magnetic resonance in clinically suspected cardiac amyloidosis: noninvasive imaging compared to endomyocardial biopsy. J Am Coll Cardiol 2008;51(10):1022–30.

45. Maceira AM, Prasad SK, Hawkins PN, et al. Cardiovascular magnetic resonance and prognosis in cardiac amyloidosis. J Cardiovasc Magn Reson 2008;10:54.

46. Dungu JN, Valencia O, Pinney JH, et al. CMR-based differentiation of AL and ATTR cardiac amyloidosis. JACC Cardiovasc Imaging 2014;7(2):133–42.

47. Mongeon FP, Jerosch-Herold M, Coelho-Filho OR, et al. Quantification of extracellular matrix expansion by CMR in infiltrative heart disease. JACC Cardiovasc Imaging 2012;5(9):897–907.

48. White JA, Kim HW, Shah D, et al. CMR imaging with rapid visual T1 assessment predicts mortality in patients suspected of cardiac amyloidosis. JACC Cardiovasc Imaging 2014;7(2):143–56.

49. Friedrich MG, Sechtem U, Schulz-Menger J, et al. Cardiovascular magnetic resonance in myocarditis: a JACC white paper. J Am Coll Cardiol 2009;53(17):1475–87.

50. Mahrholdt H. Cardiovascular magnetic resonance assessment of human myocarditis: a comparison to histology and molecular pathology. Circulation 2004;109(10):1250–8.

51. Mahrholdt H, Wagner A, Deluigi CC, et al. Presentation, patterns of myocardial damage, and clinical course of viral myocarditis. Circulation 2006; 114(15):1581–90.

52. Grun S, Schumm J, Greulich S, et al. Long-term follow-up of biopsy-proven viral myocarditis: predictors of mortality and incomplete recovery. J Am Coll Cardiol 2012;59(18):1604–15.

53. Kindermann I, Barth C, Mahfoud F, et al. Update on myocarditis. J Am Coll Cardiol 2012;59(9):779–92.

54. Ferreira VM, Piechnik SK, Dall'Armellina E, et al. T(1) mapping for the diagnosis of acute myocarditis using CMR: comparison to T2-weighted and late gadolinium enhanced imaging. JACC Cardiovasc Imaging 2013;6(10):1048–58.

55. Schumm J, Greulich S, Sechtem U, et al. T1 mapping as new diagnostic technique in a case of acute onset of biopsy-proven viral myocarditis. Clin Res Cardiol 2014;103(5):405–8.

56. Croisille P, Kim HW, Kim RJ. Controversies in cardiovascular MR imaging: T2-weighted imaging should not be used to delineate the area at risk in ischemic myocardial injury. Radiology 2012; 265(1):12–22.

57. Higgins CB, Herfkens R, Lipton MJ, et al. Nuclear magnetic resonance imaging of acute myocardial infarction in dogs: alterations in magnetic relaxation times. Am J Cardiol 1983;52(1):184–8.

58. Kim RJ, Fieno DS, Parrish TB, et al. Relationship of MRI delayed contrast enhancement to irreversible injury, infarct age, and contractile function. Circulation 1999;100(19):1992–2002.

59. Kim RJ, Wu E, Rafael A, et al. The use of contrast-enhanced magnetic resonance imaging to identify reversible myocardial dysfunction. N Engl J Med 2000;343(20):1445–53.

60. Messroghli DR, Walters K, Plein S, et al. Myocardial T1 mapping: application to patients with acute and chronic myocardial infarction. Magn Reson Med 2007;58(1):34–40.

61. Chan W, Duffy SJ, White DA, et al. Acute left ventricular remodeling following myocardial infarction: coupling of regional healing with remote extracellular matrix expansion. JACC Cardiovasc Imaging 2012;5(9):884–93.

62. Wong TC, Piehler K, Meier CG, et al. Association between extracellular matrix expansion quantified by cardiovascular magnetic resonance and short-term mortality. Circulation 2012;126(10):1206–16.

63. Moon JC, Treibel TA, Schelbert EB. T1 mapping for diffuse myocardial fibrosis: a key biomarker in cardiac disease? J Am Coll Cardiol 2013;62(14):1288–9.

Advances in MR Imaging Assessment of Adults with Congenital Heart Disease

Nazima N. Kathiria, DO*, Charles B. Higgins, MD,
Karen G. Ordovas, MD, MAS

KEYWORDS

- Congenital heart disease • Complex congenital cardiac disease • 4D flow • Ventricular strain
- Delayed enhancement • T1 mapping • 3D cardiac model • Tetralogy of fallot

KEY POINTS

- Novel MR imaging techniques for the assessment of patients with congenital heart disease include 4-dimensional flow imaging, myocardial strain imaging, tissue characterization tools, and 3-dimensional modeling.
- Current clinical research publications highlight potential applications for these techniques in the near future.

INTRODUCTION

Cardiac MR imaging is a well-established method for the diagnosis and follow-up of adult patients with congenital heart disease (CHD).[1] One of the primary roles of MR imaging in these patients is in the postoperative assessment and guidance for the timing of reintervention. Recent advances in cardiac MR imaging have the potential to increase the scope of clinical applications in these patients, expanding its role for not only diagnosis and follow-up but also risk stratification.

In this review, recent work on novel cardiac MR imaging methods in adult patients with CHD is emphasized.

NEW CLINICAL APPLICATIONS
Flow Imaging

Velocity-encoded cine MR imaging is a robust technique used clinically for the quantification of blood flow. In patients with CHD, the main application of this technique is to quantify regurgitant volumes and estimate the severity of cardiac shunts.

The development of 4-dimensional (4D) flow imaging has many potential applications in adult patients with CHD. The technique consists of a comprehensive evaluation of vascular hemodynamics, achieved through the combined data acquisition of 3 spatial dimensions and 3 blood flow velocity directions during the cardiac cycle.

Recent work from Hope and colleagues[2,3] focused on the application of 4D flow imaging in patients with coarctation of the aorta and bicuspid aortic valve. The authors showed that the quantification of collateral flow in patients with hemodynamically significant coarctation can be accurately obtained with 4D-flow imaging, using 2-dimensional (2D) flow techniques as the standard of reference.[2] In addition to providing comparable collateral flow quantification to 2D flow technique, the 4D flow approach allows for a more comprehensive evaluation of the thoracic aorta flow, including assessment of aortic valve dynamics and estimation of associated aortic valve stenosis owing to bicuspid aortic valve. Finally, the 3-dimensional (3D) acquisition allows for repositioning of the flow measurement planes

The authors have nothing to disclose.
Department of Radiology, Cardiac and Pulmonary Imaging, University of California, San Francisco, 505 Parnassus Avenue, San Francisco, CA 94143-0628, USA
* Corresponding author.
E-mail address: nnkathiria@yahoo.com

Magn Reson Imaging Clin N Am 23 (2015) 35–40
http://dx.doi.org/10.1016/j.mric.2014.09.005
1064-9689/15/$ – see front matter Published by Elsevier Inc.

during the postprocessing analysis, unlike the standard 2D flow technique.[2]

Additional applications of 4D flow in patients with CHD have been investigated. A general advantage of the method is to allow for quantification of blood flow in multiple vessels with single acquisition. Therefore, patients with complex CHD can have a mapping of the venous and arterial blood flow obtained in a timely manner.[4] Meadows and colleagues[5] successfully used the single-acquisition 4D approach to evaluate differential pulmonary flow, pulmonary regurgitation, and pulmonary stenosis in patients with tetralogy of Fallot (TOF). Four-dimensional technique permits evaluation of multiple vessels with a single acquisition and allows for the alteration of planes of choice during the postprocessing phase, unlike with 2D flow technique. These characteristics suggest added value for 4D flow imaging in clinical evaluation of patients with CHD.

The main limitations for widespread clinical applications of 4D flow include time-consuming data collection and analysis and limited spatial resolution for flow analysis in smaller vessels. The development of optimized fast sequences using sparse sampling techniques shows promise in decreasing scan time and improving spatial resolution.[6]

Quantification of Ventricular Mechanics

In current clinical practice, steady-state free precession (SSFP) cine images are the most useful sequences for qualitative and quantitative assessment of ventricular function. Volumetric analysis of SSFP images, usually obtained in the short-axis plane, permit quantification of ventricular volumes and ejection fractions. Furthermore, regional function can be quantified by measuring ventricular wall thickening during the cardiac cycle. Advanced techniques for quantification of regional myocardial strain have the potential to identify myocardial dysfunction before depression of global measures of ventricular contractility, such as ejection fraction. Different methods have been proposed for quantification of myocardial strain, which is usually measured in 3 components: circumferential, longitudinal, and radial strain.[7]

Applications of myocardial strain imaging in patients with CHD have been a recent focus of clinical research. Ordovas and colleagues[8] described how MR imaging tagging (**Fig. 1**) can aid in the early detection of left ventricular dysfunction in patients with pulmonary regurgitation after repair of TOF and normal left ventricular ejection fraction and pulmonary regurgitation after repair of TOF. The authors showed that patients with TOF have significantly decreased left ventricular peak circumferential strain in the base and apex levels compared with normal volunteers. Moreover, the left ventricular peak rotation at the basilar and midventricular levels was also delayed in these patients compared with volunteers. Additionally, the same investigators used SSFP cine sequences for quantification of ventricular septal excursion in patients after repair of TOF (**Fig. 2**). Abnormal ventricular septal excursion was associated with reduced global and septal left ventricular systolic function. It also corresponded with the presence of fibrosis at the left ventricular septum and at the right and left ventricular hinge points, suggesting the technique may be able to identify adverse interventricular interaction.[9]

Further applications of strain imaging in CHD include the assessment of ventricle-ventricle interaction such as in patients with a single right ventricle. Fogel and colleagues[10] compared single right ventricles with systemic right ventricles and found significant differences in regional wall motion and strain in single ventricle physiology depending whether a left ventricle was present to augment function. Additionally, Young and colleagues described the directionally dependent changes in strain in postaortic coarctation repair patients. They found that subjects with an increased ejection fraction also had increased strain in the circumferential direction and decreased strain in the longitudinal direction, suggesting that the elevated ejection fraction may be related to myocardial hypertrophy.[7]

Scar Imaging

Delayed gadolinium enhancement sequences have become a common tool in the evaluation of ischemic and nonischemic cardiomyopathies. Furthermore, it is an extremely useful prognostic tool in some CHDs, particularly in TOF. Babu-Narayan and colleagues[11] studied 92 adult patients after TOF repair using delayed enhancement imaging. They determined that delayed enhancement is commonly seen within the right ventricular outflow tract and ventricular septal defect patch sites but may also involve the inferior right ventricle insertion point and the left ventricle. The delayed enhancement seen within the right and left ventricles in these patients correlated with increased age, impaired exercise capacity, ventricular dysfunction, and cardiac arrhythmias.[1] These findings may be helpful in guiding management, such as timing for reintervention or need for ablation to treat and prevent arrhythmias.

Other forms of CHD are found to have delayed enhancement after surgery, including single

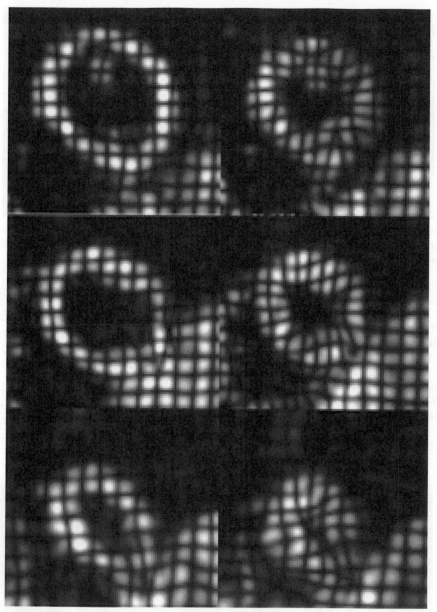

Fig. 1. Tagging acquisition of a patient with TOF at end-diastole (*left*) and end-systole (*right*) at 3 separate levels from cranial (*top*) to caudal (*bottom*).

ventricle post-Norwood procedure, which is typically within the aortic homograft.[12] However, additional studies on clinical relevance of abnormal delayed enhancement in CHD other than TOF remain to be determined.

T1 mapping is another, more recent, novel technique for myocardial tissue characterization. Regional fibrosis can be precisely identified with delayed enhancement imaging; however, diffuse myocardial fibrosis can also be assessed through calculation of the global T1 relaxation time and extracellular volume.[13,14]

Broberg and colleagues[13] compared the right and left ventricular volumes and the ejection fraction to evaluate for diffuse left ventricular fibrosis in 50 adult patients with CHD. Fibrosis values were significantly elevated in patients with CHD compared with normal controls. Diffuse fibrosis was highest in single right ventricle patients and cyanotic patients. Also, a relationship was found between ventricular end-diastolic volume and function. These findings could be useful for prognostic characterization of patients with CHD.

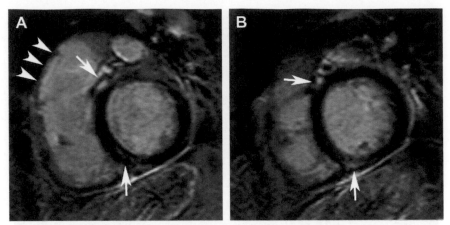

Fig. 2. Patients after repair of TOF. Delayed enhancement images in the short axis plane at the right ventricular outflow tract (RVOT) level (*A*) and midventricular level (*B*). Note the abnormal enhancement along the RVOT (*arrowheads*), and in the anterior and inferior ventricular junction points (*arrows*).

Although T1 mapping and evaluation of the extracellular volume seem promising clinically, the technique is still challenging given the variability of T1 values between scanners and different sequences used for its quantification. Moreover, larger clinical trials are necessary for confident correlations of the findings between diffuse fibrosis values and the outcomes of patients with CHD.[13,14]

3-Dimensional Models

Challenges in surgical correction of patients with complex CHDs have led to growing interest in the cardiology community for tools to help facilitate the preoperative planning, such as with 3D plastic models of the heart. Three-dimensional cardiac specimens from computed tomography and MR imaging is a cutting-edge tool that can assist the cardiac surgeon with planning before

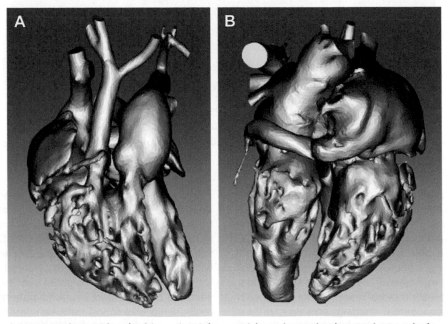

Fig. 3. Complex CHD patient with a double outlet right ventricle and upstairs-downstairs ventricular relationship. Virtual interactive 3D model reconstructed from a gadolinium enhancement MR angiography in an anterior (*A*) and posterior (*B*) projection.

the correction of complex CHD. Another potential application is to inform interventionalists on the selection of stents and catheters that would be the most effective for correction of various cardiac lesions.

The cardiac models may be created as a virtual 3D structure that allows for interactive manipulation (**Fig. 3**). Alternatively, these 3D models can be printed to provide tangible depiction of the cardiac anatomy and potentially more precise planning of the surgical correction approach, by using stored computed tomography or MR images as a stereolithography file. Using a 3D Cartesian coordinate system, the printer creates a specimen using a mixture of fluid-binding substances and ink. Layer upon layer of plaster powder is placed to create the predetermined regions of interest in the heart.[15]

Dr Yoo[16] has 2 years of clinical experience creating 3D plastic cardiac models for the preoperative assessment of patients with double outlet right ventricle. They suggest that this technology be expanded to produce cardiac models to permit practice procedures in patients with complex anatomy. In addition, it should encompass models of various surgical pathways such as Fontan and right ventricle to pulmonary artery conduit to further assess flow through complicated postsurgical pathways. Also, they believe a collection of teaching phantoms, including normal and pathologic cardiovascular anatomy, should be created. Finally, they suggest that the technique should eventually be enhanced to combine imaging data from multiple modalities.[16]

Although building 3D cardiac models of complex CHD has tremendous potential to facilitate surgical and interventional approaches for the treatment of complex CHD, the technique still has limitations. One of the primary limitations of the technique is that it is costly to generate printed heart models. In addition, it is time consuming to generate the data and then create the phantoms. Furthermore, sometimes the texture and flexibility of the material used to make the 3D model are not satisfactory to simulate the human heart and great vessels.[17]

SUMMARY

Advanced cardiac MR techniques for myocardial tissue characterization, flow evaluation, myocardial strain analysis, and 3D modeling have been recently used for assessment of adult patients after repair of CHD. Although these methods are being used mostly in the research arena, several potential diagnostic and prognostic applications are suggested.

REFERENCES

1. Kilner PJ. Imaging congenital heart disease in adults. Br J Radiol 2011;84(Spec No 3):S258–68.
2. Hope MD, Meadows AK, Hope TA, et al. Clinical evaluation of aortic coarctation with 4D flow MR imaging. J Magn Reson Imaging 2010;31(3):711–8.
3. Hope MD, Hope TA, Crooke SE, et al. 4D flow CMR in assessment of valve-related ascending aortic disease. JACC Cardiovasc Imaging 2011;4(7): 781–7.
4. Francois CJ, Srinivasan S, Schiebler ML, et al. 4D cardiovascular magnetic resonance velocity mapping of alterations of right heart flow patterns and main pulmonary artery hemodynamics in tetralogy of Fallot. J Cardiovasc Magn Reson 2012;14:16.
5. Meadows AK, Hope MD, Saloner D, et al. 4D flow for accurate assessment of differential pulmonary arterial flow in patients with tetralogy of Fallot, in 12th Annual SCMR Scientific Session. Journal of Cardiovascular Magnetic Resonance; January 28, 2009.
6. Markl M, Frydrychowicz A, Kozerke S, et al. 4D flow MRI. J Magn Reson Imaging 2012;36(5):1015–36.
7. Augustine D, Lewandowski AJ, Lazdam M, et al. Global and regional left ventricular myocardial deformation measures by magnetic resonance feature tracking in healthy volunteers: comparison with tagging and relevance of gender. J Cardiovasc Magn Reson 2013;15:8.
8. Ordovas KG, Carlsson M, Lease KE, et al. Impaired regional left ventricular strain after repair of tetralogy of Fallot. J Magn Reson Imaging 2012; 35(1):79–85.
9. Muzzarelli S, Ordovas KG, Cannavale G, et al. Tetralogy of Fallot: impact of the excursion of the interventricular septum on left ventricular systolic function and fibrosis after surgical repair. Radiology 2011;259(2):375–83.
10. Fogel MA. A study in ventricular-ventricular interaction. Single right ventricles compared with systemic right ventricles in a dual-chamber circulation. Circulation 1995;92(2):219–30.
11. Babu-Narayan SV. Ventricular fibrosis suggested by cardiovascular magnetic resonance in adults with repaired tetralogy of fallot and its relationship to adverse markers of clinical outcome. Circulation 2006;113(3):405–13.
12. Harris MA. Delayed-enhancement cardiovascular magnetic resonance identifies fibrous tissue in children after surgery for congenital heart disease. J Thorac Cardiovasc Surg 2007;133(3):676–81.
13. Broberg CS. Quantification of diffuse myocardial fibrosis and its association with myocardial dysfunction in congenital heart disease. Circ Cardiovasc Imaging 2010;3(6):727–34.
14. Moon JC. Myocardial T1 mapping and extracellular volume quantification: a Society for Cardiovascular

Magnetic Resonance (SCMR) and CMR Working Group of the European Society of Cardiology consensus statement. J Cardiovasc Magn Reson 2013;15:92.

15. Greil GF. Stereolithographic reproduction of complex cardiac morphology based on high spatial resolution imaging. Clin Res Cardiol 2007;96(3): 176–85.

16. Thabit O, Yoo SJ. Rapid prototyping of cardiac models: current utilization and future directions. J Cardiovasc Magn Reson 2012;14:T13.

17. Abdel-Sayed S, von Segesser LK. Rapid prototyping for training purposes in cardiovascular surgery. In: Hoque M, editor. Advanced applications of rapid prototyping technology in modern engineering. Rijeka, Croatia: In Tech; 2011. p. 1–15.

MR of Multi-Organ Involvement in the Metabolic Syndrome

Maurice B. Bizino, MD[a],*, Michael L. Sala, MD[a],
Paul de Heer, MSc[b], Pieternel van der Tol, MSc[a],
Jan W.A. Smit, MD, PhD[c], Andrew G. Webb, PhD[b],
Albert de Roos, MD, PhD[a], Hildebrandus J. Lamb, MD, PhD[a]

KEYWORDS

- Metabolic syndrome • Magnetic resonance imaging • Magnetic resonance spectroscopy
- Fat imaging • Nonalcoholic fatty liver disease • Diabetic cardiomyopathy
- Microstructural brain damage • Ectopic lipid accumulation

KEY POINTS

- State-of-the-art magnetic resonance (MR) technologies provide whole-body assessment of metabolic syndrome (MetS) pathophysiology and complications.
- MRI and MR spectroscopy image and quantify ectopic lipid accumulation, such as pericardial/perivascular fat, visceral abdominal fat, and fatty infiltration of organs, associated with adverse outcome.
- By using MR elastography, T1-mapping, phosphorus MR spectroscopy, and diffusion-weighted imaging, MR can assist in staging nonalcoholic fatty liver disease.
- Using cardiac MRI, spectroscopy, and mapping techniques, key features of diabetic cardiomyopathy, such as diastolic dysfunction, left ventricular hypertrophy, myocardial steatosis and fibrosis, can be quantified.
- Novel MR techniques, such as magnetization transfer imaging and diffusion tensor imaging, demonstrate microstructural brain damage in MetS.

INTRODUCTION
Epidemiology

About one third of the United States population of 20 years or older has metabolic syndrome (MetS) and its prevalence increases with advancing age and body mass index,[1] stressing its tight association with the obesity epidemic.

Definition

Diagnosis of MetS requires positive identification of at least 3 out of 5 criteria displayed in **Table 1**. As

such, approximately 90% of type 2 diabetes mellitus (DM2) patients have MetS.[1] Patients with MetS are heterogeneous in nature with varying risk of disease and consequently require personalized care, for example, by MR prognosis, in terms of future cardiovascular and cerebrovascular events (**Fig. 1**).[2]

MRI of Multi-Organ Involvement in the Metabolic Syndrome

MetS is a systemic disease with complex pathophysiology including insulin resistance,

The authors have nothing to disclose.
[a] Department of Radiology, Leiden University Medical Center, Albinusdreef 2, Leiden 2333 ZA, The Netherlands; [b] C.J. Gorter Center for High Field MRI, Department of Radiology, Leiden University Medical Center, Albinusdreef 2, Leiden 2333 ZA, The Netherlands; [c] Division of Endocrinology, Department of Medicine, Radboud University Medical Centre, PO Box 9101, 6500 HB, Nijmegen, The Netherlands
* Corresponding author. Albinusdreef 2, postzone C3Q, Leiden 2333 ZA, The Netherlands.
E-mail address: m.b.bizino@lumc.nl

Table 1
Diagnosis of MetS

MetS Criteria (NCEP-ATP III Criteria)	Definition
Abdominal obesity: waist circumference	Men >40 inches Women >35 inches
Increased plasma triglyceride level	>150 mg/dL
Decreased plasma HDL level	Men <40 mg/dL Women <50 mg/dL
Elevated blood pressure	>130/85 mm Hg
Increased plasma fasting glucose	>100 mg/dL

Three out of five criteria are necessary for the diagnosis.
  Abbreviations: HDL, high-density lipoprotein; MetS, metabolic syndrome; NCEP-ATP III, National Cholesterol and Education Program – Adult Treatment Panel III.
  From National Heart, Lung, and Blood Institute. Third report of the expert panel on detection, evaluation, and treatment of high blood cholesterol in adults. Bethesda (MD): National Heart, Lung, and Blood Institute; 2002. NIH publication number 02-5215.

atherogenic dyslipidemia, hypertension, ectopic lipid accumulation, low-grade inflammation, prothrombotic state, and fibrosis resulting in end-organ damage.[3] MRI and magnetic resonance spectroscopy (MRS) can be used to quantify ectopic lipid accumulation. Importantly, as shown in **Fig. 2**, functional and structural consequences of MetS can be evaluated with MR on a whole-body level. In the liver, several techniques—ranging from MRS and water fat imaging to magnetic resonance elastography (MRE) and T1 mapping—are used to quantify hepatic steatosis and differentiate between stages of nonalcoholic fatty liver disease (NAFLD). In parallel, cardiac MR can quantify myocardial steatosis and associated complications, such as diastolic dysfunction and fibrosis. In the brain, magnetization transfer imaging and diffusion tensor imaging (DTI) can detect microstructural brain damage associated with MetS. The involvement of various other organs ranging from kidney to pancreas and skeletal muscle can be assessed with MR.

Purpose of Review

This review highlights MR techniques that assess multi-organ involvement in MetS.

ADIPOSE TISSUE
White Adipose Tissue

Abdominal visceral obesity
Ectopic lipid accumulation in white adipose tissue (WAT) predominantly occurs in the visceral abdominal compartment. Visceral white adipocytes can contribute to MetS etiology by secreting excessive amounts of plasma free fatty acids, adipokines, and cytokines. MetS prevalence correlates with waist circumference, reflecting the role of abdominal obesity. However, waist circumference does not differentiate between subcutaneous adipose tissue (SAT) and visceral adipose tissue (VAT). Given that VAT has a stronger association with MetS than SAT, differentiation between SAT and VAT is critical.[3] Several MR techniques can be used to reliably quantify SAT and VAT. These include T1-weighted imaging, frequency-selective lipid imaging, and chemical shift-encoded water–fat imaging, all different methods that can be lumped under the umbrella of water–fat MRI (**Figs. 3** and **4**). An appropriate sequence can be chosen on the basis of local accessibility, available scanning time, and presence of image postprocessing expertise. An overview of MR techniques for lipid quantification and their advantages/disadvantages is reviewed by Hu and Kan.[4]

Pericardial and perivascular fat
In addition to abdominal VAT, ectopic lipid accumulation around the heart (pericardial fat) and vessels (perivascular fat) is increased in MetS. Pericardial/perivascular fat is physiologically protective in terms of mechanical support and as a source of biochemical substrates, hormones, and cytokines. However, increased pericardial/perivascular lipid accumulation in MetS has been linked with low-grade systemic inflammation, adverse metabolic profile and risk of ischemic heart disease.[5] Various electrocardiogram-gated MR sequences, including steady-state free precession short axis sequences, fat-selective imaging (see **Fig. 4**), and water–fat MRI, can be used to image pericardial fat and enable volume quantification in a reproducible manner.[1]

Brown Adipose Tissue

In contrast to WAT, brown adipose tissue (BAT) volume and activity are diminished in obesity and may play a role in its development. BAT contributes significantly to total resting energy expenditure by dissipating glucose and free fatty acids into heat. The reference method for imaging BAT volume and activity is fluorodeoxyglucose PET-CT after mild cold exposure. The desire for a nonirradiating alternative has led to many MR techniques being evaluated to image BAT. These techniques identify BAT by its higher water fraction compared with WAT. However, MR of BAT is limited by the fact that, in humans, BAT and WAT are not entirely separated anatomically, complicating reliable BAT volume quantification. MRI

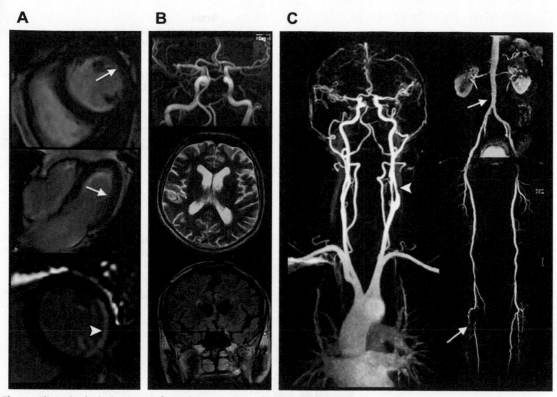

Fig. 1. Clinical whole-body MR for risk estimation of future cardiovascular events. Images acquired in a 74-year-old man with a 21-year history of type 2 diabetes mellitus. (*A*) Cardiac MRI involving cine imaging (*top* and *middle*) showing hypokinesia in the anterolateral segment (*arrow*). The bottom image is a late gadolinium-enhanced image displaying subendocardial enhancement (*arrowhead*) consistent with myocardial infarction. (*B*) Cerebral arteries using time-of-flight angiography (*top*), an axial T2-weighted brain image (*middle*) and a coronal fluid-attenuated inversion-recovery image (*bottom*). These images show no overt brain abnormalities associated with the metabolic syndrome (MetS). (*C*) Contrast-enhanced MR angiograms of carotid arteries (*left*) and abdominal and lower extremity arteries (*right*) with *arrowhead* and *arrows* indicating stenosis owing to atherosclerotic disease. Using this 60-minute MR protocol, future cardiac and cerebrovascular events can be predicted in DM patients with higher accuracy compared with clinical characteristics.[1] (*From* Bamberg F, Parhofer KG, Lochner E, et al. Diabetes mellitus: long-term prognostic value of whole-body MR imaging for the occurrence of cardiac and cerebrovascular events. Radiology 2013;269(3):733, with permission.)

of BAT activity is still in its infancy, although promising results using T2* imaging have been published recently.[4]

LIVER
Hepatic Steatosis

Ectopic lipid accumulation in the liver, that is, hepatic steatosis, is present in the majority of MetS patients and plays a central role in the pathogenesis of insulin resistance, hyperglycemia, and atherogenic dyslipidemia. The gold standard to determine hepatic steatosis is histology which requires a biopsy. However, several MR techniques can assess hepatic triglyceride (TG) content noninvasively with lower sampling error.[1]

Currently, proton MRS (^{1}H-MRS) is the noninvasive gold standard to quantify hepatic TG content

(**Fig. 5**). ^{1}H-MRS has the best sensitivity for detection of small amounts of fat. A drawback of this technique is the risk of sampling error inherent to quantifying TG content in a small voxel.

Recently, the mDIXON technique using multiple echoes has been shown to enable liver fat quantification (**Fig. 6**). By applying the mDIXON technique, T2* effects caused by the relatively high iron content in the liver can be compensated. The technique is becoming increasingly popular because of its advantages of small sampling error (because it is a whole-organ imaging technique) and fast data acquisition.

Multidimensional chemical shift imaging is a multivoxel ^{1}H-MRS technique that measures a grid of multiple voxels, thus reducing sampling error. The disadvantage of chemical shift imaging is that data acquisition is slow and technically challenging.

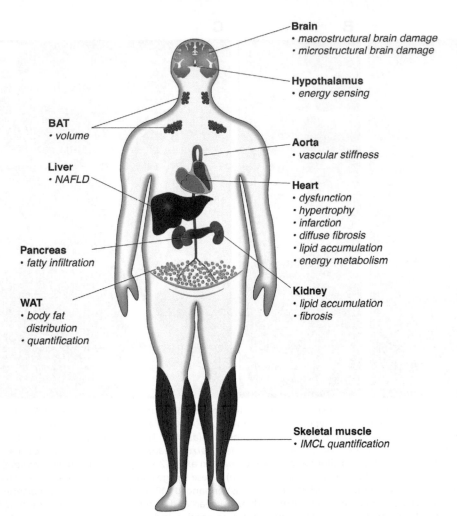

Fig. 2. Overview of MR assessment of multi-organ involvement in metabolic syndrome. Key features of multi-organ involvement in the metabolic syndrome (MetS) that can be assessed with MR are shown. MRI accurately assesses the distribution of WAT showing abundance of visceral adipose tissue (VAT) and peri-organ adipose tissue. In contrast, brown adipose tissue volume is diminished in obesity, suggesting that diminished thermogenesis may be involved in the etiology of MetS. Excessive accumulation of triglycerides in the liver, that is, hepatic steatosis, may play a central role in the development of MetS. Hepatic steatosis can progress into nonalcoholic steatohepatitis (NASH), fibrosis, and cirrhosis. Both excessive VAT and hepatic steatosis are strongly linked to insulin resistance, a key component of MetS. The cardiovascular system can be involved focally (eg, myocardial infarction) or globally (eg, diabetic cardiomyopathy). Cardiac remodeling of the cardiovascular system involves the sequelae of fatty infiltration, inflammation, fibrosis, and ultimately organ failure. Furthermore, brain involvement in MetS is increasingly being studied. In addition to macrostructural changes, such as brain atrophy and cerebral small vessel disease, microstructural changes are important features of MetS brain pathology. Various other organs, such as the kidney, pancreas, and skeletal muscle, undergo pathologic alterations in MetS patients. BAT, brown adipose tissue; WAT, white adipose tissue.

Progression of Hepatic Steatosis into Inflammation, Fibrosis, and Cirrhosis

Hepatic steatosis can progress into nonalcoholic steatohepatitis, fibrosis, and ultimately cirrhosis and hepatic failure, a disease spectrum termed NAFLD. MRE, T1 mapping, phosphorus MRS (^{31}P-MRS), and diffusion-weighted imaging (DWI) are the focus of ongoing research to differentiate

between NAFLD stages, and explore potential advantages compared with histology, that is, lower sampling error and fewer complications.[6]

MRE (**Fig. 7**) is an emerging technique that quantitatively images shear waves in the liver produced by external mechanical waves. A few validation studies have shown MRE's capability of differentiating between stages of NAFLD.[7]

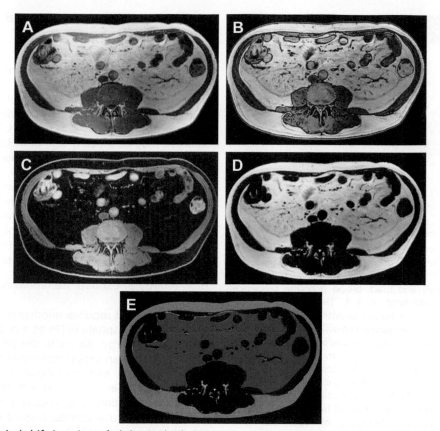

Fig. 3. Chemical shift imaging of abdominal adipose tissue and subsequent volume quantification. Transverse slice at the level of L5 vertebra acquired with an mDIXON method using 2 echoes, (*A*) 1 in-phase and (*B*) 1 out-of-phase image. From these images, (*C*) a water image and (*D*) fat image can be reconstructed. (*E*) Image post processing can be used to semiautomatically assess subcutaneous (*green*) and visceral (*red*) adipose tissue. This sequence was performed in a patient with longstanding type 2 diabetes mellitus showing relatively large amounts of visceral adipose tissue compared with subcutaneous adipose tissue.

T1 mapping is more readily available than MRE in terms of commercially available imaging sequences. This technique is based on the increased T1 relaxation time of edematous (nonalcoholic steatohepatitis) and fibrotic tissue. In NAFLD, several studies have been performed, showing a strong correlation between increasing T1 and increasing stages of fibrosis (see **Fig. 7**).[8] In parallel with quantification of extracellular volume (ECV) expansion in cardiac imaging, ECV quantification in the liver is also feasible.[9] However, validation studies for ECV mapping to quantify liver fibrosis have yet to be published.

^{31}P-MRS can quantify metabolites involved in cell membrane metabolism as well as regulators of fibrosis pathogenesis can be assessed (**Fig. 8**). Additionally, hepatic energy metabolism can be assessed by quantifying high energy phosphates.[10]

DWI is a promising technique that measures water movement in extracellular space. Unfortunately, DWI is less reliable in the presence of fat, which limits its use in NAFLD. Future studies must focus on correcting for the influence of fat in order for DWI to become suitable for NAFLD staging.[6]

HEART

Cardiac MRI (anatomic, functional, angiography, perfusion, late gadolinium enhancement) is an important component in the assessment of a major complication of MetS, namely ischemic heart disease, which is reviewed elsewhere.[11] This section covers MR techniques to assess nonischemic remodeling in MetS, that is, "diabetic cardiomyopathy," which is characterized by diastolic dysfunction, hypertrophy, disrupted cardiac energy metabolism, and ECV expansion related to myocardial fibrosis.

Diastolic Dysfunction

Diastole comprises a combination of active (energy-consuming) relaxation and passive

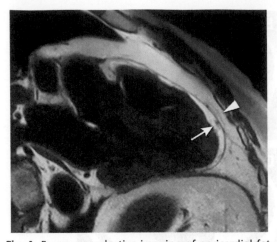

Fig. 4. Frequency selective imaging of pericardial fat. Three-chamber view acquired with a turbo spin echo sequence with a spectral presaturation with inversion recovery (SPIR) and black blood prepulse sequence during 1 breath-hold at 3 T. This high-resolution sequence enables separate quantification of epicardial (*arrow*) and paracardial (*arrowhead*) fat volumes. Note the high paracardial fat mass in this male patient with type 2 diabetes mellitus. In addition to their different anatomic relation to coronary arteries, epicardial and paracardial fat have a different embryonic origin; epicardial fat has brown adipose tissue characteristics, whereas the paracardial fat does not. Therefore, separate quantification of epicardial and paracardial fat could reveal varying effects on end-organ damage.

compliance. In MetS, diastolic dysfunction is an early feature and independent predictor of mortality. Diastolic dysfunction is caused by altered myocardial energetics and by diminished ventricular compliance.[1] MR using phase contrast imaging with velocity encoding is a robust technique to quantitatively assess diastolic function (**Fig. 9**). Although the left ventricle (LV) has been the primary focus of research, recent findings show that right ventricular diastolic dysfunction is analogous to LV diastolic dysfunction.[12]

Hypertrophy

LV end-diastolic mass-to-volume ratio is tightly linked to markers of insulin resistance, indicating concentric LV remodeling in MetS.[11] **Fig. 9** shows an example of LV mass quantification with MR.

Cardiac Energy Metabolism

Cardiac energy metabolism is crucial for both systolic and diastolic function. As such, alterations in myocardial energetics may constitute the first step in heart failure pathophysiology.[13] MRS enables

in vivo quantification of myocardial energetics (**Fig. 10**).

Myocardial steatosis

An increased storage of TG in cardiomyocytes is a hallmark of diabetic cardiomyopathy.[1] As shown in animal studies, increased storage of myocardial TG reflects an abundance of toxic lipids that impair cardiomyocyte integrity and function. Myocardial steatosis may be an early sign of diabetic cardiomyopathy, because it is an independent predictor of diastolic dysfunction. Importantly, myocardial steatosis and diastolic dysfunction are reversible, signifying a window of opportunity for therapeutic interventions aimed at preventing overt heart failure.[1] MR is the only modality capable of quantifying myocardial TG content. **Fig. 11** shows an example of cardiac ^{1}H-MRS spectroscopy.

High-energy phosphate metabolism: fuel for function

The human heart requires enormous amounts of adenosine triphosphate (ATP) as a primary carrier of chemical energy. As such, the phosphocreatine/ATP ratio is an important indicator of cardiac energy reserve and metabolic efficiency. A decreased ratio is associated with diastolic and systolic dysfunction. The finding that, in DM2 patients with normal cardiac mass and function, the phosphocreatine/ATP ratio was decreased compared with healthy controls, reflects the possibility that disruptions in myocardial energetics might play a role in the pathogenesis of cardiomyopathies.[13] **Fig. 12** shows an example of ^{31}P-MRS of the heart. Up to now, the use of cardiac ^{31}P-MRS has been limited to a research setting in experienced centers because of its complex acquisition.

Extracellular Volume Expansion

Another hallmark of diabetic cardiomyopathy is ECV expansion caused by collagen deposition, referred to as myocardial fibrosis. Fibrosis is associated with mortality and activation of the renin–angiotensin–aldosterone system[11] and can be quantified using a modified Look Locker (MOLLI) or shortened MOLLI sequence.[14,15] Using these sequences, native T1 mapping and postcontrast T1 mapping can be performed. By combining these images, fractional ECV can be quantified (**Fig. 13**).

BRAIN INVOLVEMENT IN THE METABOLIC SYNDROME
Brain Structures Involved in Feeding Behavior

Multiple brain structures are functionally involved in the regulation of food intake. Homeostatic

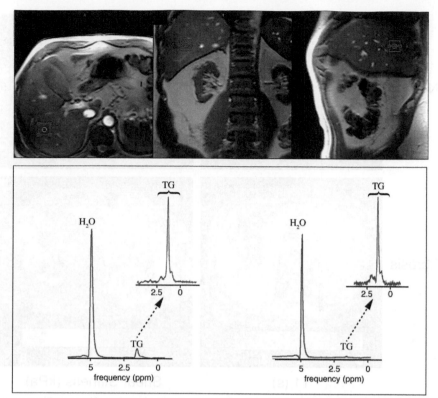

Fig. 5. Proton magnetic resonance spectroscopy (^{1}H-MRS) of the liver to quantify hepatic triglyceride content. Voxel planning and examples of proton spectra acquired from the liver at 3 T. ^{1}H-MRS is based on the fact that different molecules have different chemical environments that translate to small differences in the strength of the magnetic field for the different metabolites. This effect is commonly known as chemical shift. In the recorded spectrum, the difference in magnetic field results in different resonance frequencies, expressed in parts per million (ppm) with respect to that of tetrametylsilane, for the various metabolites. In practice, 1 spectra without water suppression is recorded to use as an internal reference, and 1 or more with water suppression are acquired for quantification of triglycerides (TG). To be able to measure small metabolite levels, it is necessary to measure a volume much larger than the normal pixel size in MRI. *Upper panel*, Typical 8-mL voxel for liver ^{1}H-MRS. *Lower panel*, Acquired unsuppressed and water-suppressed spectra of an obese (*left*) and lean (*right*) volunteer. In liver spectra, TG is mainly represented by 3 different proton moieties, namely, CH_2-CH = CH-CH_2, (-CH_2)$_n$, and -CH_3. To quantify the fat percentage often the integrals below the (-CH_2)$_n$ and CH_3 peaks are summed and divided by the sum of the integrals of the water and (-CH_2)$_n$ and CH_3 peaks. In this example, the calculated hepatic triglyceride content was 8.26% for the obese subject and 1.24% for the lean subject.

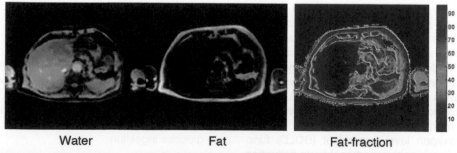

Fig. 6. DIXON MRI of the liver to quantify hepatic triglyceride content. The *left* and *middle images* are the reconstructed water and fat images, respectively. A 6-point DIXON sequence was used with a starting echo time of 0.74 ms and echo spacing of 1 ms. The fat fraction was calculated on a pixel-by-pixel basis by dividing the fat image by the sum of the water and fat image. For this obese subject, the calculated fat fraction was between 3% and 9%, depending on the location, illustrating the inhomogeneous nature of hepatic steatosis.

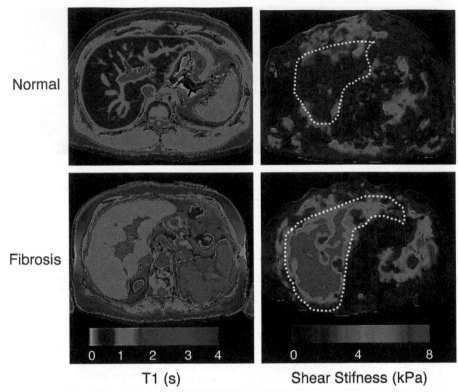

Normal

Fibrosis

T1 (s)   Shear Stifness (kPa)

Fig. 7. Magnetic resonance elastography and T1 mapping: Quantitative imaging of hepatic fibrosis in nonalcoholic fatty liver disease (NAFLD). Examples of T1 mapping (*left*) and magnetic resonance elastography (MRE; *right*) in healthy versus fibrotic liver tissue (as assessed by biopsy). T1 maps were acquired with a shortened modified Look Locker (shMOLLI) sequence in a single breath-hold. Increasing T1 values were correlated with increasing degrees of fibrosis. MRE is performed using mechanical waves transmitted by an acoustic pressure driver. Using automated post processing, data are translated into quantitative images displaying tissue shear stiffness in kPa. It has been shown that MRE is a useful tool to detect advanced stages of fibrosis. The dotted lines indicate the liver. (*From* [*Left*] Banerjee R, Pavlides M, Tunnicliffe EM, et al. Multiparametric magnetic resonance for the non-invasive diagnosis of liver disease. J Hepatol 2014;60(1):72, with permission; and [*right*] Kim D, Kim WR, Talwalkar JA, et al. Advanced fibrosis in nonalcoholic fatty liver disease: noninvasive assessment with MR elastography. Radiology 2013;268(2):415, with permission.)

regulation of food intake is driven by inputs from the basal ganglia, thalamus, and hippocampus. Interestingly, a recent study found increased amygdalar and hippocampal volumes, as assessed by 3-dimensional T1-weighted MRI, in elderly obese individuals.[16] The finding that these morphometric changes occurred in the amygdala and hippocampus but not in other brain structures that play a role in feeding behavior suggests that cognitive aspects may be of major importance in the regulation of feeding.[16] Additional studies are required to examine the mechanisms behind the observed morphometric changes.

Blood oxygen level–dependent (BOLD) functional MRI is a sensitive marker of brain activation. It has been shown previously that healthy, lean volunteers demonstrated a significant dose-dependent decrease of the BOLD signal in the hypothalamus after glucose ingestion.[17] In patients with DM2, hypothalamic neuronal activity is altered, as demonstrated by the absence of a BOLD signal decrease after glucose ingestion.[18] Recently it has been shown that after following a very low-calorie diet for 4 days, the hypothalamus in DM2 patients responds to glucose ingestion similarly to that in healthy subjects.[19] Because the hypothalamus is involved in the control of postprandial metabolism, this may explain the strong metabolic improvement that can be observed in DM2 patients upon caloric restriction.[19] Future studies are needed to elucidate the fundamental mechanisms behind the hypothalamic response to glucose ingestion.

Structural Brain Damage

Although cardiovascular disease is considered to be the main long-term complication of MetS,

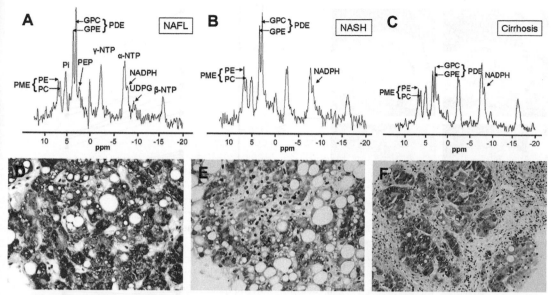

Fig. 8. Phosphorus magnetic resonance spectroscopy (^{31}P-MRS) of the liver to differentiate between simple steatosis, steatohepatitis, and cirrhosis. *Upper panel (A–C)*, ^{31}P spectra, acquired at 3 T, of simple steatosis (nonalcoholic fatty liver [NAFL]), nonalcoholic steatohepatitis (NASH), and cirrhosis, respectively. This technique quantifies markers of hepatocyte membrane integrity. Corresponding liver biopsy specimens are shown in the *lower panel (D–F)*. The ratio of NADPH/(PME + PDE) was significantly lower in NAFL compared with NASH and cirrhosis, whereas the ratios of PE/(PME + PDE) and GPC/(PME + PDE) were higher in cirrhosis compared with NASH and NAFL. GPC, glycerophosphocholine; GPE, glycerophosphosrylethanolamine; NADPH, nicotinamide adenine dinucleotide phosphate; NTP, nucleoside triphosphate; PC, phophoscholine; PDE, phosphodiester; PE, phosphosethanolamine; PEP, phosphoenolpyruvate; Pi, inorganic phosphate; PME, phosphomonoester; UDPG, uridine diphosphosglucose. (*From* Sevastianova K, Hakkarainen A, Kotronen A, et al. Nonalcoholic fatty liver disease: detection of elevated nicotinamide adenine dinucleotide phosphate with in vivo 3-T 31P MR spectroscopy with proton decoupling. Radiology 2010;256(2):472; with permission.)

multiple organs may be affected, including the brain.[1] Risk factors associated with MetS accelerate cerebral small vessel disease, which may result in white matter lesions, cerebral microbleeds, and brain atrophy, as detected by conventional structural MRI.[20] Subtle microstructural brain damage may occur in the normal appearing brain tissue in the absence of overt brain abnormalities.[21]

DTI is an MRI technique that is well suited to detect early microstructural changes in normal-appearing brain tissue in a number of disease states. Using DTI, Shimoji and colleagues[22] recently found that fractional anisotropy (FA) values were lower in MetS subjects relative to control subjects. FA reflects the "coherence" of highly structured tissue, such as axon bundles. Accordingly, lower FA values indicate microstructural brain tissue decline. Regional brain analysis showed that mean FA values of the right inferior fronto-occipital fasciculus were lower in MetS subjects compared with controls subjects.[22] The inferior fronto-occipital fasciculus connects all 4 major lobes of the brain and may play an important role in linking all the components of what is commonly referred to as the social brain. The social brain hypothesis may in turn be related to human feeding behavior; several functional MRI studies have detected a correlation between neural activity and eating behavior.

Magnetization transfer imaging is another sensitive MRI technique that can be used to evaluate changes in brain microstructure.[23] Using both DTI and magnetization transfer imaging, Sala and colleagues[21] recently showed that clustering of risk factors in MetS is associated with evidence of microstructural damage in the gray and white matter as indicated by a decreased magnetization transfer ratio histogram peak height and increased mean diffusivity. Voxel-wise analysis of cortical gray matter magnetization transfer ratio showed that changes were diffuse and symmetric in both hemispheres. Future longitudinal studies should determine whether these changes evolve into more pronounced structural deterioration or changes in cognition.

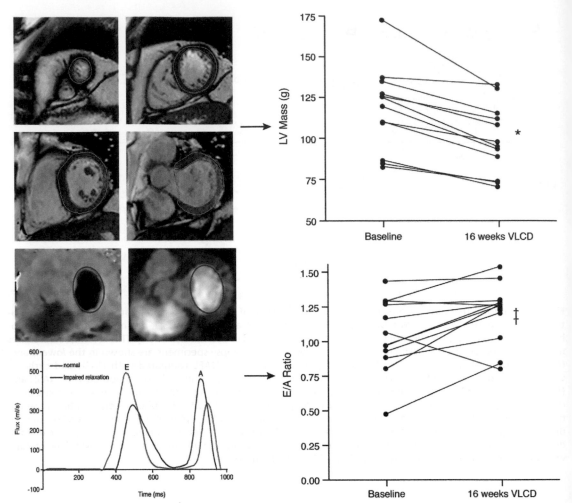

Fig. 9. Reversible cardiac manifestations in metabolic syndrome: hypertrophy and diastolic dysfunction. MR measures left ventricular (LV) mass and diastolic function reliably and quantitatively, enabling detection of, for example, the effects of nutritional interventions in relatively small study populations. The *upper left panel* shows manual segmentation of myocardium in end-diastolic shorts axis images. Using dedicated software, LV mass can be calculated, showing that LV mass diminished in all type 2 diabetes mellitus patients after a 16-week very low-calorie diet (VLCD). Decreased LV mass was tightly linked with improved diastolic function as reflected by an improved E/A ratio (E = early filling phase, A = atrial late filling phase). This parameter can be measured by using phase contrast MR with velocity encoding (*lower right panel*). By acquiring a 2-dimensional acquisition plane centered on the atrioventricular valve, a time–velocity or time–flow rate curve can be generated. Recent studies have shown an increased reliability of diastolic function assessment using 3-dimensional 3-directional velocity encoding with retrospective tracking to compensate for valve movement and changing flow direction throughout the cardiac cycle. * $P<.001$; † $P<.05$. (From [*Left lower panel*] van der Meer RW, Lamb HJ, Smit JW, et al. MR imaging evaluation of cardiovascular risk in metabolic syndrome. Radiology 2012;264(1):31, with permission; and [*Right panel*] Hammer S, Snel M, Lamb HJ, et al. Prolonged caloric restriction in obese patients with type 2 diabetes mellitus decreases myocardial triglyceride content and improves myocardial function. J Am Coll Cardiol 2008;52(12):1011, with permission.)

Arterial Stiffness

Pulse wave velocity (PWV) is a surrogate marker of vascular stiffness. It is defined as the velocity of the systolic wave front propagating through the vessels (**Fig. 14**) with increased PWV, indicating arterial wall stiffening. MRI enables PWV assessment in different vascular territories, including the aortic arch and the carotid arteries. By using MRI, Roes and colleagues[24] found that aortic PWV was increased in MetS subjects. Another study found that aortic PWV is associated with LV mass and lacunar brain infarcts in hypertensive patients.[25] These observations may be

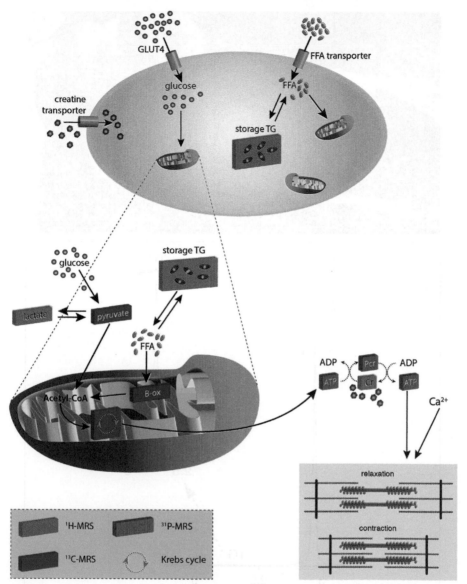

Fig. 10. MR spectroscopy assessment of cardiac energy metabolism. The cardiomyocyte is represented in orange. FFAs and glucose, in a ratio of 3:1, are the primary sources of chemical energy for the production of ATP, which takes plays in the mitochondrion (*blue*). FFAs are either stored as TGs or oxidized (B-ox) to give acetyl-CoA. Glucose is glycolysed—in the presence of oxygen—to pyruvate, another substrate for acetyl-CoA, which enters the Krebs cycle for oxidative phosphorylation. This process provides energy required to form ATP. In the mitochondrion, ATP and Cr give rise to phosphocreatine (PCr), which diffuses to the myofibril, where it is converted into mechanical energy, under tight control of the Ca^{2+} flux. Note here that both systole and diastole require ATP. The colored boxes (*yellow, green,* and *red*) indicate opportunities for measurement with ¹H, ³¹P and ¹³C MRS, respectively. For ¹H and ³¹P, see also **Figs. 15** and **16**. Cardiac ¹³C-MRS has not yet been performed in humans, but animal studies using hyperpolarized metabolic tracers have shown the feasibility of using cardiac ¹³C-MRS to assess fuel flux (B-ox, Krebs cycle, pyruvate). Acetyl-CoA, acetyl-coenzyme A; ADP, adenosine diphosphate; ATP, adenosine triphosphate; B-ox, β-oxidation; Ca^{2+}, ionized calcium; Cr, creatine; FFA, free fatty acid; GLUT4, glucose transporter type 4; PCr, phosphocreatine; TG, triglyceride content. (*From* Bizino MB, Hammer S, Lamb HJ. Metabolic imaging of the human heart: clinical application of magnetic resonance spectroscopy. Heart 2014;100(11):881–90; with permission.)

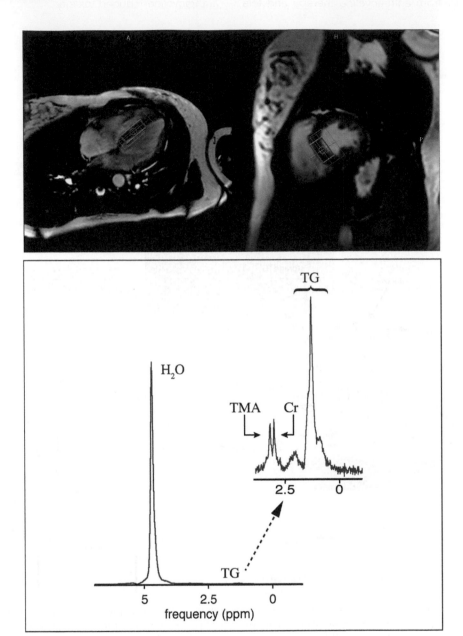

Fig. 11. Cardiac proton magnetic resonance spectroscopy (^{1}H-MRS) to quantify myocardial steatosis. Cardiac ^{1}H-MRS was performed on 1.5 and 3 T MR systems using commercially available transceiver coils, and recently at 7 T using custom-built detectors. Cardiac ^{1}H-MRS is subject to motion artifacts owing to contraction and breathing. To overcome these issues, cardiac ^{1}H-MRS is usually performed with electrocardiographic gating and either breath-holding or free breathing with respiratory motion triggering/compensation. To prevent contamination of pericardial fat, the voxel of interest (VOI) is placed in the interventricular septum. The most commonly used pulse sequences are stimulated echo acquisition mode (STEAM) and point resolved spectroscopy (PRESS). The low abundance of the various metabolites requires water suppression and acquisition of multiple averages resulting in relatively long scan duration. The water-suppressed spectrum displayed in the lower panel shows signals from creatine (Cr), triglycerides (TG) and trimethyl ammonium (TMA). In this example, 16 non–water-suppressed and 48 water-suppressed averages were acquired at 3 T from a VOI of 15 mL.

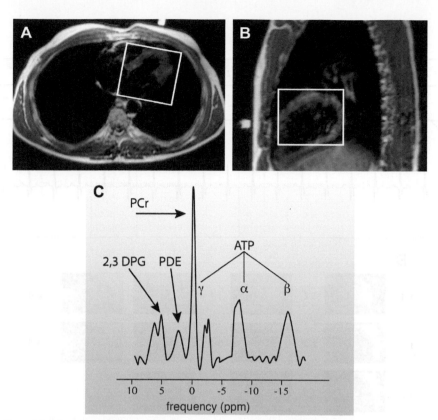

Fig. 12. Cardiac phosphorus magnetic resonance spectroscopy (^{31}P-MRS) to assess high-energy phosphates. Cardiac ^{31}P-MRS at 1.5 T is performed by positioning a volume of interest (*square box*) over almost the entire heart (*A, B*); eliminating signal contamination from skeletal muscle is essential. The PCr/ATP ratio can be calculated from the spectrum (*C*) and is an important representation of cardiac energy reserve. In the metabolic syndrome (MetS), a decreased PCr/ATP ratio has been found before the onset of overt heart failure. ATP, adenosine triphosphate; 2,3 DPG, 2,3-diphosphglycerate; PCr, phosphocreatine; PDE, phosphodiesters; ppm, parts per million. (*From* Bizino MB, Hammer S, Lamb HJ. Metabolic imaging of the human heart: clinical application of magnetic resonance spectroscopy. Heart 2014;100(11):881–90; with permission.)

explained by the concept that aortic stiffening increases exposure of the microcirculation to abnormal physical forces that may lead to end-organ damage.[26] MRI enables a comprehensive evaluation of the heart, large vessels, and brain. Future studies should focus on the pathogenesis of end-organ damage in MetS, and evaluate the effect of interventions.

OTHER ORGANS
Kidney

The relationship between MetS and chronic kidney disease (CKD) has become increasingly clear over the past years. Even before the onset of overt diabetes or hypertension, patients have an increased risk of microalbuminuria and renal insufficiency. CKD pathophysiology involves accumulation of toxic lipids, inflammation, neurohumoral factors, and ultimately fibrosis.[27] MR assessment of renal TG content (RTGC) was performed in diabetic mice, using chemical shift-selective imaging in combination with BOLD MRI. The results showed that RTGC was inversely correlated with intrarenal oxygenation, suggesting a possible causal link between RTGC and CKD.[28] Recently, it has been shown that human RTGC can be assessed reliably with ^{1}H-MRS (**Fig. 15**).[29] Therefore, renal ^{1}H-MRS provides a tool to study the association between RTGC, MetS, and CKD in humans. As a final common pathway of CKD in MetS, quantitative imaging of renal fibrosis—in parallel with heart and liver—with MR is an obvious next step. To this end, several methods, such as quantitative susceptibility mapping and renal T1 mapping, are promising.[30]

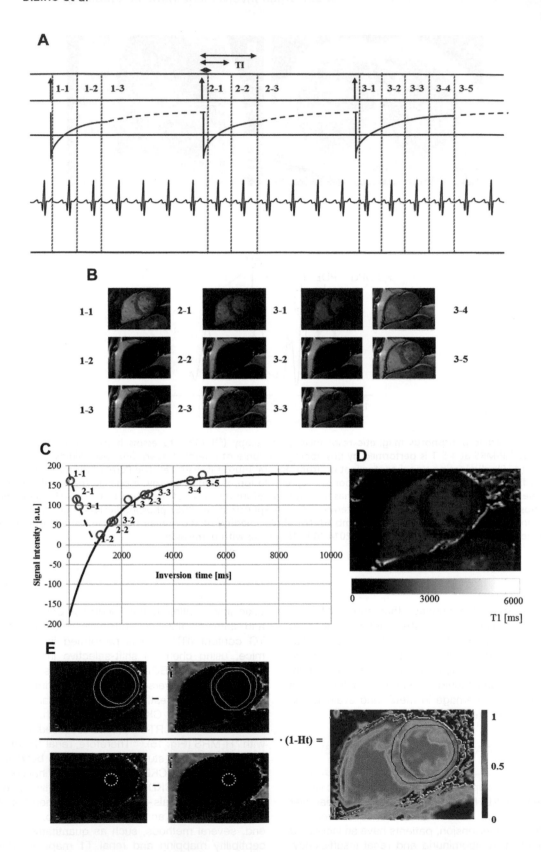

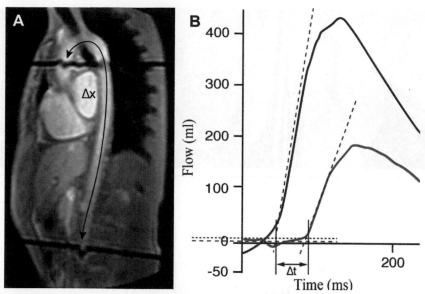

Fig. 14. MR assessment of arterial stiffness: Pulse wave velocity (PWV). Through-plane velocity encoded MRI assessment of PWV at 1.5 T. (*A*) Sagittal gradient-echo image aligned with the long axis of the aorta shows 2 perpendicular image acquisition planes through the ascending aorta and abdominal aorta. The path length is indicated by *Δx*. (*B*) Velocity curves are used to assess the time delay (*Δt*) of the arrival of the proximal (*blue curve*) and abdominal flow (*red curve*). The PWV is calculated as *Δx/Δt*.

Pancreas

In parallel with NAFLD, fatty pancreas is associated with visceral obesity and hypertriglyceridemia. This was shown in a population study using iterative decomposition of water and fat with echo asymmetry and least squares estimation (IDEAL), which is a DIXON-based technique with 3 echoes to account for both B0 and B1 magnetic field inhomogeneities.[31] Further studies are needed to clarify the role of fatty pancreas in MetS pathophysiology.

Fig. 13. MR acquisition and image after processing to evaluate fibrosis in diabetic cardiomyopathy. Modified Look Locker inversion recovery (MOLLI) sequence to determine T1 values of myocardium and subsequent use of precontrast and postcontrast T1 maps to calculate extracellular volume, acquired at 3 T. (*A*) The MOLLI experiment. This technique consists of 3 consecutive electrocardiogram triggered look locker (LL) experiments, with a three (1), three (2), and five (3) segment single-shot readout. Between each LL experiment, 4 heartbeats are used for magnetization recovery. (*B, C*) In total, within a 17–heart-beat breath-hold, the longitudinal relaxation curve is sampled at 11 different inversion times. The images are reordered based on increasing inversion time, that is, the time between the inversion pulse and the readout. (*D*) The T1 map can be calculated by performing voxel wise fitting the signal intensity (SI): $SI[a.u.] = A - B \times e^{-TI/T_1}$, $T_1 = T_1^*((B/A) - 1)$. A commonly used variation on the MOLLI method is the shortened MOLLI (ShMOLLI), where only 2 consecutive electrocardiograph-triggered LL experiments are performed with a 5 and 1 single shot read out. (*E*) The formula used to calculate the extracellular volume fraction (ECV): $ECV_{myo} = \frac{(R_{1,post,myo} - R_{1,pre,myo})}{(R_{1,post,blood} - R_{1,pre,blood})} (1 - Ht)$. The ECV is determined with a combination of native and postcontrast T1 mapping. The gadolinium-based contrast agent will distribute in the extracellular space of the myocardium. Therefore, a higher concentration of gadolinium indicates a larger ECV, which could indicate more fibrosis. In the example given in this figure, acquired in a 66-year-old type 2 diabetes mellitus patient with myocardial infarction, the average ECV of the myocardium was 0.34, or 34%, compared with 27% in healthy volunteers.

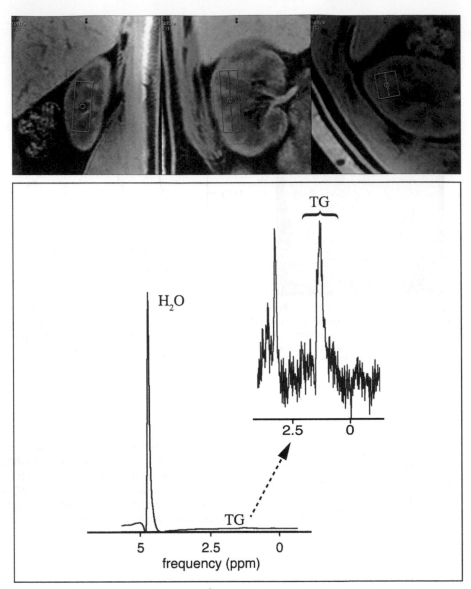

Fig. 15. Proton magnetic resonance spectroscopy (^{1}H-MRS) for the evaluation of renal steatosis. MR spectra of the kidney at 3 T. Sixteen water spectra and 64 water-suppressed breath-hold spectra were acquired with a PRESS sequence from a 4-mL voxel. The renal fat fraction in this healthy volunteer was 0.28%. Compared with liver, lipid levels are lower, and also owing to the smaller organ size, the voxel of interest (VOI) must be smaller; both result in lower signal-to-noise ratio (SNR) in the kidney, requiring greater signal averaging. TG, triglycerides; ppm, parts per million.

Skeletal Muscle

An increased level of intramyocellular lipids, without a corresponding increase in extramyocellular lipids, is a key feature of peripheral insulin resistance, that may play a role in the increased hepatic steatosis and dyslipidemia, observed in MetS.[32,33] ^{1}H-MRS is the only technique sensitive enough to differentiate intramyocellular lipids from extramyocellular lipids (**Fig. 16**). Using ^{31}P-MRS, skeletal muscle phosphate–ATP flux can be assessed, thereby providing insight into mitochondrial (dys)function and its relationship with insulin sensitivity.[34]

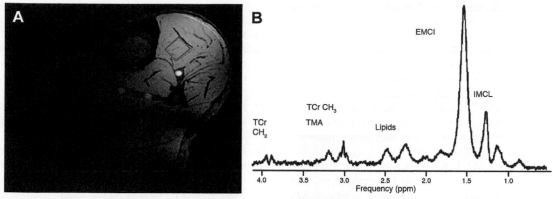

Fig. 16. Skeletal muscle proton magnetic resonance spectroscopy (^{1}H-MRS) at 7 T. (*A*) The *red box* shows the voxel of interest in the tibialis anterior muscle of a healthy volunteer scanned on a 7 T system. (*B*) The corresponding ^{1}H spectrum shows clear separation of intramyocellular lipids (IMCL) and extramyocellular lipids (EMCL). IMCL is strongly linked to insulin resistance, whereas EMCL is not. Other peak assignments: tCr, total creatine (CH2 and CH3 resonances); TMA, tri-methyl ammonium.

SUMMARY

MR is a powerful, noninvasive tool to assess multi-organ involvement in MetS. Key elements of MetS pathophysiology, ranging from ectopic lipid accumulation to end-organ damage of liver, heart, brain, kidney, pancreas, and skeletal muscle, can be evaluated using a multitude of MR techniques. As such, MR has proven its utility with respect to unraveling MetS pathophysiology, as well as monitoring efficacy of therapeutic interventions.

ACKNOWLEDGMENT

The authors thank G. Kracht for figure composition and layout.

REFERENCES

1. van der Meer RW, Lamb HJ, Smit JW, et al. MR imaging evaluation of cardiovascular risk in metabolic syndrome. Radiology 2012;264(1):21–37.

2. Bamberg F, Parhofer KG, Lochner E, et al. Diabetes mellitus: long-term prognostic value of whole-body MR imaging for the occurrence of cardiac and cerebrovascular events. Radiology 2013;269(3):730–7.

3. Despres JP, Lemieux I. Abdominal obesity and metabolic syndrome. Nature 2006;444(7121):881–7.

4. Hu HH, Kan HE. Quantitative proton MR techniques for measuring fat. NMR Biomed 2013; 26(12):1609–29.

5. Iozzo P. Myocardial, perivascular, and epicardial fat. Diabetes Care 2011;34(Suppl 2):S371–9.

6. Cobbold JF, Patel D, Taylor-Robinson SD. Assessment of inflammation and fibrosis in non-alcoholic fatty liver disease by imaging-based techniques. J Gastroenterol Hepatol 2012;27(8):1281–92.

7. Kim D, Kim WR, Talwalkar JA, et al. Advanced fibrosis in nonalcoholic fatty liver disease: noninvasive assessment with MR elastography. Radiology 2013;268(2):411–9.

8. Banerjee R, Pavlides M, Tunnicliffe EM, et al. Multi-parametric magnetic resonance for the non-invasive diagnosis of liver disease. J Hepatol 2014; 60(1):69–77.

9. Bandula S, Banypersad SM, Sado D, et al. Measurement of Tissue interstitial volume in healthy patients and those with amyloidosis with equilibrium contrast-enhanced MR imaging. Radiology 2013; 268(3):858–64.

10. Sevastianova K, Hakkarainen A, Kotronen A, et al. Nonalcoholic fatty liver disease: detection of elevated nicotinamide adenine dinucleotide phosphate with in vivo 3-T 31P MR spectroscopy with proton decoupling. Radiology 2010;256(2):466–73.

11. Shah RV, Abbasi SA, Kwong RY. Role of cardiac MRI in diabetes. Curr Cardiol Rep 2014;16(2):449.

12. Widya RL, van der Meer RW, Smit JW, et al. Right ventricular involvement in diabetic cardiomyopathy. Diabetes Care 2013;36(2):457–62.

13. Bizino MB, Hammer S, Lamb HJ. Metabolic imaging of the human heart: clinical application of magnetic resonance spectroscopy. Heart 2014; 100(11):881–90.

14. Messroghli DR, Radjenovic A, Kozerke S, et al. Modified look-locker inversion recovery (MOLLI) for high-resolution T1 mapping of the heart. Magn Reson Med 2004;52(1):141–6.

15. Piechnik SK, Ferreira VM, Dall'Armellina E, et al. Shortened modified look-locker inversion recovery (ShMOLLI) for clinical myocardial T1-mapping at 1.5 and 3 T within a 9 heartbeat breathhold. J Cardiovasc Magn Reson 2010;12:69.

16. Widya RL, de Roos A, Trompet S, et al. Increased amygdalar and hippocampal volumes in elderly obese individuals with or at risk of cardiovascular disease. Am J Clin Nutr 2011;93(6):1190–5.

17. Smeets PA, de GC, Stafleu A, et al. Functional MRI of human hypothalamic responses following glucose ingestion. Neuroimage 2005;24(2):363–8.

18. Vidarsdottir S, Smeets PA, Eichelsheim DL, et al. Glucose ingestion fails to inhibit hypothalamic neuronal activity in patients with type 2 diabetes. Diabetes 2007;56(10):2547–50.

19. Teeuwisse WM, Widya RL, Paulides M, et al. Short-term caloric restriction normalizes hypothalamic neuronal responsiveness to glucose ingestion in patients with type 2 diabetes. Diabetes 2012;61(12):3255–9.

20. Kloppenborg RP, Nederkoorn PJ, Grool AM, et al. Cerebral small-vessel disease and progression of brain atrophy: the SMART-MR study. Neurology 2012;79(20):2029–36.

21. Sala M, de RA, Berg AV, et al. Microstructural brain tissue damage in metabolic syndrome. Diabetes Care 2014;37(2):493–500.

22. Shimoji K, Abe O, Uka T, et al. White matter alteration in metabolic syndrome: diffusion tensor analysis. Diabetes Care 2013;36(3):696–700.

23. Seiler S, Cavalieri M, Schmidt R. Vascular cognitive impairment - an ill-defined concept with the need to define its vascular component. J Neurol Sci 2012;322(1–2):11–6.

24. Roes SD, Alizadeh DR, Westenberg JJ, et al. Assessment of aortic pulse wave velocity and cardiac diastolic function in subjects with and without the metabolic syndrome: HDL cholesterol is independently associated with cardiovascular function. Diabetes Care 2008;31(7):1442–4.

25. Brandts A, van Elderen SG, Westenberg JJ, et al. Association of aortic arch pulse wave velocity with left ventricular mass and lacunar brain infarcts in hypertensive patients: assessment with MR imaging. Radiology 2009;253(3):681–8.

26. Mitchell GF, van Buchem MA, Sigurdsson S, et al. Arterial stiffness, pressure and flow pulsatility and brain structure and function: the age, gene/environment susceptibility – Reykjavik study. Brain 2011; 134(Pt 11):3398–407.

27. Singh AK, Kari JA. Metabolic syndrome and chronic kidney disease. Curr Opin Nephrol Hypertens 2013; 22(2):198–203.

28. Peng XG, Bai YY, Fang F, et al. Renal lipids and oxygenation in diabetic mice: noninvasive quantification with MR imaging. Radiology 2013;269(3): 748–57.

29. Hammer S, de Vries AP, de Heer P, et al. Metabolic imaging of human kidney triglyceride content: reproducibility of proton magnetic resonance spectroscopy. PLoS One 2013;8(4):e62209.

30. Xie L, Sparks MA, Li W, et al. Quantitative susceptibility mapping of kidney inflammation and fibrosis in type 1 angiotensin receptor-deficient mice. NMR Biomed 2013;26(12):1853–63.

31. Wong VW, Wong GL, Yeung DK, et al. Fatty pancreas, insulin resistance, and beta-cell function: a population study using fat-water magnetic resonance imaging. Am J Gastroenterol 2014;109(4): 589–97.

32. Flannery C, Dufour S, Rabol R, et al. Skeletal muscle insulin resistance promotes increased hepatic de novo lipogenesis, hyperlipidemia, and hepatic steatosis in the elderly. Diabetes 2012;61(11):2711–7.

33. Boesch C, Machann J, Vermathen P, et al. Role of proton MR for the study of muscle lipid metabolism. NMR Biomed 2006;19:968–88.

34. Kemp GJ, Brindle KM. What do magnetic resonance-based measurements of Pi – ATP flux tell us about skeletal muscle metabolism? Diabetes 2012;61:1927–34.

MR Safety Issues Particular to Women

Pierluigi Ciet, MD[a,b,c], Diana E. Litmanovich, MD[a],*

KEYWORDS

- Pregnancy • IUD • Fetal • Cardiovascular • MR

KEY POINTS

- MR imaging has been increasingly used in cardiovascular imaging, especially in young women and during pregnancy, because of the lack of ionizing radiation.
- Cardiovascular MR scan of women poses gender-specific risks, such as those related to pregnancy, lactation, and use of intrauterine devices.
- To date, there is no evidence on the short-term and long-term adverse effects of the static magnetic field on human health.
- The American College of Radiology Guidance Document on MR Safe Practices (2013) states that pregnant patients should undergo MR imaging only if (1) the required information cannot be obtained via other nonionizing means, (2) the information is likely to alter patient care, and (3) the examination cannot wait until after completion of the pregnancy.
- At present, there is no scientific evidence contraindicating MR imaging in women bearing intrauterine devices.

INTRODUCTION

Magnetic Resonance (MR) imaging has been increasingly used in cardiopulmonary imaging, especially in young women and during pregnancy[1] because cardiopulmonary disorders can affect up to 4% of all pregnancies in the industrialized world because of preexisting conditions or conditions acquired during pregnancy.[1] The increased use of MR imaging for cardiovascular imaging in woman is mainly caused by the lack of ionizing radiation, which has made this technique preferable to computed tomography (CT).[1] However, MR has general hazards related to the use of magnetic fields, which can be categorized as static, pulsed radiofrequency (RF), and time-varying gradient electromagnetic fields.[2] The hazards for large

static magnetic fields are the biological effects, projectile effect, and implant/monitoring device malfunction and/or displacement.[2] The RF pulses pose problems of tissue and implant heating.[2] For time-varying gradient electromagnetic fields, the hazards are mainly peripheral nerve stimulation and acoustic noise.[2] These general MR hazards are routinely addressed by MR safety procedures, which are applied to prevent and reduce risk. However, there are also specific female gender–related MR hazards, which can be of concern for radiologists, MR technicians, and ordering physicians.

This article focuses on familiarizing radiologists with MR safety issues and current, evidence-based recommendations for pregnant or lactating women and for women who have intrauterine

The authors have nothing to disclose.
[a] Department of Radiology, Beth Israel Deaconess Medical Center, 330 Brookline Avenue, Boston, MA 02215, USA; [b] Department of Radiology, Erasmus Medical Center, Postbus 2040, 3000 CA, Rotterdam, The Netherlands; [c] Department of Pediatrics, Respiratory Medicine and Allergy, Erasmus Medical Center-Sophia Children's Hospital, Wytemaweg 80, 3015 CN, Rotterdam, The Netherlands
* Corresponding author.
E-mail address: dlitmano@bidmc.harvard.edu

Magn Reson Imaging Clin N Am 23 (2015) 59–67
http://dx.doi.org/10.1016/j.mric.2014.09.002
1064-9689/15/$ – see front matter © 2015 Elsevier Inc. All rights reserved.

devices (IUDs) in place. Practical algorithms to minimize risk and increase MR safety for women are also suggested.

General Safety Aspects of MR Imaging: Potential Generic Hazards in MR Imaging

The MR system uses 3 types of magnetic fields simultaneously[2]:

- Static magnetic fields (B_0)
- Time-varying magnetic field gradients
- RF magnetic fields

Effects of static magnetic fields

The static or main magnetic field is used to align the hydrogen protons in the patient's body. This strong magnetic field is always active, even when the MR scanner is not imaging. The strengths of the static magnetic fields used in clinical and research MR systems range between 1 T and 7 T. The most common systems are 1.5 T and 3 T and these represent 60% to 75% and 5% to 15% of the all MR imaging system in United States, respectively.[3]

There are 2 major safety issues related to high static magnetic field strength: attraction of ferromagnetic material toward the magnet and biological effects.[3] Any object containing ferromagnetic material is pulled toward the core of the main magnet and this is known as the projectile effect. Anyone or anything in the direct trajectory of the object can be hit by the object moving toward the magnet, with the risk of severe injuries. Patients must be screened for MR compatibility before being allowed into the MR environment (**Box 1**).[4] However, current physiologic monitoring devices, instruments, and pacemakers are made to be MR compatible, so the risk of displacement in the body is negligible.[4,5]

The biological effects of static magnetic fields are still controversial.[6] A review of the safety of high static magnetic field strength on human health concludes that there are no firmly established detrimental effects except for sensory effects, such as vertigo, metallic taste, and magnetophosphenes.[7] The International Commission on Non-Ionizing Radiation Protection (ICNIRP)[8,9] stated that there is no evidence on the short-term and long-term adverse effects of the static magnetic field on human health.

Effects of time-varying magnetic field

The function of the time-varying magnetic field gradients in an MR system is to determine position-dependent variation in magnetic field strength.[3] The main safety concerns with time-varying magnetic field gradients are related to biological effects

---

Box 1
Medical devices and materials that need to be screened for MR safety

Aneurism Clips, Carotid artery vascular clamps

Biopsy needles, markers

Breast tissue expanders and implants

Bone and spinal fusion stimulators

Cardiac pacemakers, electrocardiogram electrodes, heart valve prosthesis

Cochlear implants, hearing aids

Dental implants, devices, and materials

Tattoos and permanent make-up

Any devices that may contain ferromagnetic material

Data from Shellock FG. Reference manual for magnetic resonance safety, implants and devices. 2014 edition. Playa Del Rey (CA): Biomedical Research Publishing Group; 2014.

---

and acoustic noise.[2] Time-varying magnetic fields generate electric fields and circulating currents in conductive tissues of the human body and these induced electric currents could interfere with the normal function of nerve cells and muscle fibers. However, at the strength used in medical imaging, these effects are thought to be minimal and not harmful.[6] A second problem related to the switching on and off of the gradient is the production of a substantial amount of acoustic noise.[3] This noise is frequently described as tapping, knocking, or twitting sounds. Intensity and frequency of these noises vary accordingly to the MR imaging parameters and sequences[10] and usually increase with reductions in slice thickness, field of view, repetition time, and echo time. Temporary hearing loss has been reported using conventional sequences.[10] For this reason ear plugs or noise reduction headphones are routinely used for MR imaging examination.[11]

Effects of radiofrequency fields

RF pulses are used in MR for nuclei excitation.[3] RF pulses can interact with both tissues and any medical devices implanted in the patient. During an MR scan, a large part of RF pulse energy is transferred into the human body as heat.[12] This tissue heating is largest at the body surface and minimal at the center of the body. The dosimetric parameter used to quantify RF energy deposition is represented in terms of specific absorption ratio (SAR), which is normally measured in Watts per kilogram.[11] All MR systems monitor the level of SAR during image acquisition, and the admitted SAR is usually 4 W/kg for a whole-body scanner, calculated for a body temperature increase of up to 0.6°C and a scanning time of 20 to 30 minutes.[11] For a given pulse sequence, the SAR depends on the static magnetic field strength, flip angle, number of RF pulses during each repetition time of the sequence, and spacing between the RF pulses. An increase in the first 3 parameters and a decrease in the last parameter can all cause an increase in SAR. Three operational levels of SAR are defined by the ICNIRP[9]:

1. The normal level, which causes no physiologic stress to patients
2. The first level, which may cause physiologic stress to the patient that may need to be controlled by medical supervision
3. The second level, in which a significant patient risk may be produced and for which explicit approval is required

Note that it has been shown that, when the average whole-body SAR remains below the safety limits, hot spots can still occur; therefore the automatic control system of the scanner is not sufficient to ensure patient safety.[13] Most of the reported accidents are burns caused by hot spots in the presence of conducting materials close to the patient, such as monitoring equipment, or in patients with tattoos and permanent cosmetics made with iron oxide or other metal-based pigments.[11]

Hazard Related to Gadolinium-Based Contrast Agent Administration

Adverse reactions to gadolinium-based contrast agent (GBCA) are classified as renal and nonrenal. The main adverse renal reaction is nephrogenic systemic fibrosis (NSF), which is a serious medical condition associated with exposure to GBCAs in patients with renal insufficiency or on dialysis.[14] Because NSF only occurs in patients with impaired renal function, GBCA administration is contraindicated in patients with chronic kidney disease (glomerular filtration rate [GFR] <30 mL/min/ 1.73 m^2) and in patients with acute kidney injury according the American College of Radiology (ACR) guidelines. In patients with GFR less than 60 mL/min/1.73 m^2, a half dose of GBCAs should be considered.[14]

Nonrenal adverse reactions are mainly allergic reactions such as nausea, hives, taste disturbance, and anaphylactoid reactions. These reactions are rare, occurring in less than 0.01% of the patients.[15] Special precaution is indicated in patients with asthma or history of allergies because the likelihood of adverse reactions is higher in these groups of patients.

Safety Aspects of MR Imaging in Women

Gender-related issues that may affect MR safety include pregnancy, lactation, and the presence of IUDs.

MR imaging of pregnant patients

MR imaging is frequently used in pregnant patients when additional information is needed to guide management beyond that available with ultrasonography, which is usually the first-line imaging method. MR is preferred to CT because of the lack of ionizing radiation. Although MR imaging has not been shown to have any deleterious effects on the fetus, the safety of MR imaging during pregnancy has yet to be definitively established.[16,17] There are 3 potential hazardous effects that MR imaging can have on the fetus[12,18,19]:

1. Potential biological damage related to cell migration, proliferation, and differentiation, possibly leading to miscarriage caused by exposure to the static magnetic field
2. Tissue heating potential and secondary damage, particularly with regard to organogenesis caused by energy deposition by RF pulses
3. Potential damage to the fetal ear (especially after 24 weeks' gestation) caused by the high acoustic noise level in varying gradient electromagnetic fields, particularly with fast-acquisition sequences[10]

Although no harmful effects have been shown using diagnostic MR in pregnancy, the ACR Guidance Document on MR Safe Practices (2013) states that pregnant patients should undergo MR imaging only if (1) the required information cannot be obtained via other nonionizing means, (2) the information is likely to alter patient care, and (3) the examination cannot wait until after completion of the pregnancy.[4]

Teratogenesis The static magnetic field of MR imaging can potentially alter cell migration, proliferation, and differentiation within the fetus, resulting in teratogenesis. Most of the studies supporting this have been performed in animals and with controversial results.[12] Multiple studies in humans show no scientific evidence of teratogenesis up to 9 years after exposure to MR imaging in utero.[19] In terms of risks of MR imaging exposure, the ACR does not distinguish between the first trimester of pregnancy and the second and third trimesters.[4] As per the ACR White Paper, at any stage during pregnancy, a risk-benefit analysis should be performed before MR imaging. Because the risk of MR at 1.5 T is theoretic, if MR imaging information is needed for patient care, the risk-benefit analysis will decide in favor of performing the clinically indicated study.

Tissue heating Human embryos and fetuses are vulnerable to chemical and physical insults during defined stages of development. As described earlier, exposure to RF pulses can cause tissue heating, with subsequent heating of fetal stem cells and, as a result, potential teratogenesis.[12] The fetus is entirely dependent on maternal temperature as well as circulation to avoid hyperthermia. Spontaneous abortion and malformations in the fetus have been reported as a result of maternal fever ($\geq 37.8°C$)[20] and hot tub use.[21] In general, maternal temperature more than 2°C greater than normal for extended periods, or 2°C to 2.5°C greater than normal for 0.5 to 1 hour, have been reported in the literature as thresholds for heat-induced fetal abnormalities.[12] The incidence of these abnormalities is directly proportional to the grade of temperature increase and exposure duration. This stage of organogenesis is most susceptible to hyperthermia because of rapid cell proliferation but the time window of the organogenesis varies according the organ considered. SAR units for MR imaging are regulated by the US Food and Drug Administration (FDA), which currently makes no specific recommendations for pregnant patients.[1]

For pregnant patients, ICNIRP guidelines state that exposure duration should be reduced to the minimum and only at the normal operation level.[9] However, most heating created by MR imaging is superficial and is absorbed by the maternal body with only a fraction reaching the fetus.[18] Further, in the study by Hand and colleagues,[18] fetal SAR and fetal temperature were shown to be within international safety limits for MR imaging procedures compliant with the ICNIRP. An international consensus states that MR imaging of pregnant patients should be performed with up to 3.0 T magnets or less to minimize SAR. In summary, heating related to RF magnetic fields is unlikely to be teratogenic, but to date no epidemiologic studies are available to assess possible long-term health effects caused by these nonionizing MR radiations.[18]

Acoustic damage By 24 weeks of pregnancy, the fetal ear develops and is able to hear noise.[19] A study on noise exposure in pregnancy for the American Academy of Pediatrics found higher frequency hearing loss, shortened gestation, and decreased birth weight in the exposed group compared with the control group.[22] The effect of MR imaging noise on the fetus is of concern because pregnant women are protected by headphones or earplugs, but the fetuses are not. The MR imaging noise level can be as high as 80 to 120 dB, but the maternal body attenuates the noise substantially, by at least 30 dB. This attenuation results in less than 90 dB of noise reaching the fetal ear. It is noteworthy that 90 dB is suggested by the American Academy of Pediatrics as the upper limit beyond which permanent damage to the fetal ear might be expected.[22] To date, no scientific evidence of acoustic damage in human fetuses has been reported in association with MR imaging exposure.

Hazards Related to Intravenous Gadolinium-based Contrast Agent Administration During Pregnancy and Lactation

Gadolinium-based contrast agents during pregnancy

GBCAs injected intravenously cross the placenta by passive diffusion across the chorionic epithelium.[23] The contrast is filtered through the kidneys and subsequently excreted into the amniotic fluid through the urine. Animal studies have shown that only 0.01% of the injected gadolinium dose was present in the fetus 4 hours after contrast injection, with only traces remaining after 24 hours; however, the half-life of gadolinium in the human fetus is unknown.[24] Concern has focused on the toxic free gadolinium ion, which can be formed by dissociation of the ion from the chelating agent. Although the stability of the gadolinium-chelate complex is unknown, one study showed that, even in patients with severely reduced renal function, no free gadolinium ion could be measured in the blood on 5 consecutive days after the administration of contrast medium.[25] Gadolinium has been shown in animal studies to have teratogenic effects when administered at high and repeated doses.[23] Although no human studies have been conducted to assess the teratogenic effect of gadolinium in pregnant women, there have been no harmful events reported so far in human fetuses exposed to GBCAs in utero.[26]

In 2013, the ACR stated that GBCAs may be given to pregnant patients if needed, by joint decision of the radiologist and referring physician only when essential to the diagnosis, when no alternative imaging studies are available, and when delaying the MR imaging examination until after delivery would be impossible.[4] The FDA states that GBCA should only be administered in pregnancy if the potential benefit justifies the potential risk to the fetus.[27] No specific neonatal tests are necessary after delivery, because no adverse effects, teratogenesis, or acoustic damage have been documented in association with the use of GBCAs for medical imaging.[23]

Gadolinium-based contrast agents during lactation

Only minimal amounts of gadolinium-based contrast material are excreted through breast milk and absorbed by the infant bowel (0.01% of injected dose).[24] This expected absorbed dose is less than 0.05% of the intravenous (IV) contrast amount recommended by the American Academy of Pediatrics for neonates undergoing a gadolinium-enhanced MR imaging study.[14] Thus, as per the ACR Contrast Manual 2013, no interruption of lactation is required if IV gadolinium is administered to a nursing patient.[14] The European Medicines Agency suggests that breastfeeding should be interrupted for more than 24 hours if the mother has been injected with the 3 least thermodynamically stable GBCAs: gadodiamide (Gd-DTPA-BMA), gadoversetamide (Gd-DTPA-BMEA), or gadolinium-diethylenetriamine penta-acetic acid (Gd-DTPA).[15,23] To date, there is no evidence of adverse reactions occurring in infants who are breastfeeding from mothers previously injected with GBCAs.

MR Safety and Intrauterine Devices

MR safety in women using IUDs depends on the device structure and composition (**Fig. 1**).[28] As previously described, the presence of a metallic device in a patient undergoing MR imaging may cause injury from movement or excessive heating of the object. Moreover, metallic devices can cause imaging artifacts, which can hamper the diagnostic accuracy. These artifacts, also known as magnetic susceptibility artifacts, consist of areas of focal loss of signal, surrounded by a hyperintense halo and associated with variable degrees of surrounding tissue distortion.[29] The size and shape of the artifact depends on the size and shape, orientation, and nature of the ferromagnetic device, as well as the sequences used in the examination.[29] IUDs can consist of nonmetallic or metallic components. The nonmetallic IUDs are usually made of plastic and are combined with progesterone. These devices do not pose any risk to women during MR imaging.[28] Metallic IUDs usually contain copper (Cu), which is not ferromagnetic. The main concern in using Cu-IUDs is related to possible injuries to the endometrium or generation of imaging artifacts. Several studies have proved that Cu-IUDs are MR safe and do not produce dislocation, heating, or image artifact.[28] Another metallic gynecologic device is the Essure system (Conceptus Inc, San Carlo, CA), a sterilization method that contains 2 metallic microimplants of stainless steel, nickel, and titanium. Essure has been proved to be safe at magnetic fields up to 3T.[28] At present, there is no scientific evidence contraindicating MR imaging in women bearing gynecologic devices (**Table 1**).[28]

MEDICOLEGAL ISSUES
Risk Management

ACR guidelines for risk management in MR imaging of pregnant patients include the following:

1. A recognized algorithm for evaluating pregnant patients in a radiological facility
2. A written policy for management of pregnant and lactating women
3. Accessibility of radiologists knowledgeable in MR imaging exposure effects to patients and referring physicians
4. Documentation in the radiology report of all discussions with patients about the risks/benefits of specific MR examinations[4]

Four main questions have to be answered by the referring clinician and radiologist when planning MR imaging during pregnancy:

1. Can the information be obtained without MR imaging examinations (eg, with ultrasonography)?
2. Can the information be obtained without IV gadolinium administration?
3. Will the information obtained with imaging affect the care of the patient or fetus during the pregnancy?
4. Can imaging be safely deferred until after pregnancy?

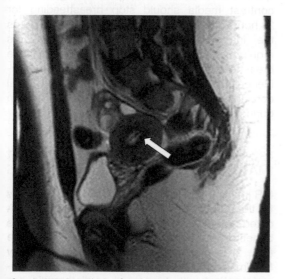

Fig. 1. MR imaging of IUD. Pelvis sagittal view, T2-weighted fast spin echo. Note the T-shaped IUD in the fundus of the uterus (*white arrow*).

Table 1
IUD and MR compatibility

Object	Status	Field Strength
Contraceptive IUD Mirena (polyethylene, barium sulfate) Berlex Laboratories, Montville, NJ	Safe	3
Contraceptive IUD Multiload Cu-375 (copper, silver) Miscellaneous (eg, Williams Medical Supply, Nashville, TN)	Safe	1.5
Contraceptive IUD Nova T (copper, silver) Miscellaneous (eg, Bayer Health Care Pharmaceuticals Inc, Whippany, NJ)	Safe	1.5
Contraceptive IUD, Copper T (copper) Miscellaneous (eg, Searle Pharmaceuticals, Chicago, IL)	Safe	1.5
Contraceptive IUD, Lippey loop, plastic Miscellaneous (eg, Skyla, Bayer HealthCare Pharmaceuticals Inc, Whippany, NJ)	Safe	1.5
Contraceptive IUD, Copper T 380A ParaGard, FEI, North Tanawanda, NY	Conditional 5	3
IUD, LCS Ultra Low Dose Levonorgestrel Contraceptive System Bayer HealthCare Pharmaceuticals Inc, Whippany, NJ	Conditional 6	3

SAFE means that the object is considered to be safe for the patient undergoing an MR procedure or an individual in the MR environment, with special reference to the highest static magnetic field strength that was used for the MR safety test.

Conditional 5 means that this object is acceptable for a patient undergoing an MR procedure or an individual in the MR environment only if specific guidelines or recommendations are followed.

Conditional 6 means that this implant/device was determined to be MR-conditional according to the terminology specified in the American Society for Testing and Materials international designation F2503: Standard Practice for Marking Medical Devices and Other Items for Safety in the Magnetic Resonance Environment.

Data from Shellock FG. Reference manual for magnetic resonance safety, implants and devices. 2014 edition. Playa Del Rey (CA): Biomedical Research Publishing Group; 2014.

Informed Consent

At our institution, informed consent is obtained for all MR imaging examinations obtained during pregnancy. While obtaining informed consent, the radiologist should explain the need for imaging and the importance of the diagnosis for the patient's care, as well as giving a brief explanation of the ordered imaging test. While summarizing the estimated risk to the patient and the fetus, the radiologist also has the opportunity to confirm the patient's comprehension of the risks and benefits as well as alternative options before consenting.[4] It is important to emphasize that there is no documented risk to the mother and the fetus caused by MR imaging.

It is important to explain to lactating patients that only a very small amount of gadolinium contrast media reaches the fetal blood when a lactating woman is given gadolinium contrast agents.[23] Thus, as per the ACR Contrast Manual 2013, no interruption of lactation is required if IV gadolinium is administered to a nursing patient.[14] In Europe, according the guidelines of the European Medicines Agency, breastfeeding should be interrupted for more than 24 hours in mothers who have been injected with the 3 least thermodynamically stable GBCAs: Gd-DTPA-BMA (@Omniscan), Gd-DTPA-BMEA (@OptiMARK), or Gd-DTPA (@Magnevist), referred to as the highest-risk agents.[15,23] Therefore, according the European guidelines, lactating women who receive the highest risk gadolinium contrast media should stop breastfeeding for 24 hours and discard the expressed milk, whereas the intermediate-risk and lowest-risk agents require discussion about whether to discontinue breastfeeding for 24 hours.[23] In summary, more evidence is needed to reach an international consensus on the problem of GBCA administration during pregnancy and lactation.

PROPOSED PRACTICAL ALGORITHMS FOR MR IMAGING SCANNING IN PREGNANT PATIENTS

MR imaging can be obtained in pregnant patients for the purposes of cardiothoracic imaging if indicated, after careful discussion of risks versus benefits with the referring clinician. Algorithm 1 (**Fig. 2**) is designed to help determine whether MR imaging is the modality of choice for the female patient with suspected cardiothoracic disease (MR imaging of pulmonary arteries, MR of peripartum cardiomyopathy).

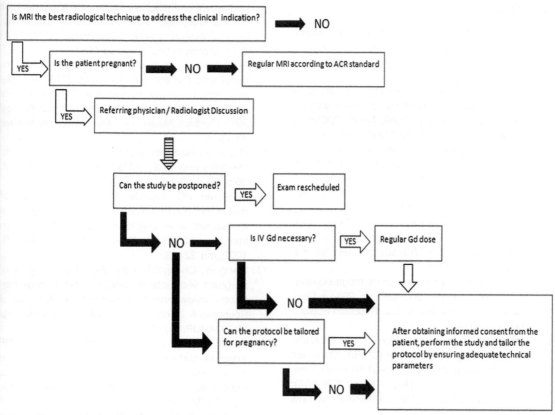

Fig. 2. Suggested approach to MR examination in pregnancy.

PRACTICAL APPROACH RELATED TO MR IMAGING PROCEDURE IN INTRAUTERINE DEVICE–BEARING WOMEN

In the MR imaging safety screening procedure, the type of IUD and its MR imaging compatibility has to be verified and documented in the safety screening form for MR imaging procedures.[4] Any complaint of pelvic pain should result in the immediate suspension of the examination.[28] In case of IUD-related discomfort during the MR imaging procedure, the patient is advised to have the correct position of the IUD checked by ultrasonography to avoid a potential unintended pregnancy resulting from dislocation. For a list of currently available IUD devices, see **Table 1**.

SUMMARY

Despite potential adverse implications of MR imaging, MR procedures are safer than any other clinical test using ionizing radiation. MR imaging retains a crucial place in a variety of potential clinical scenarios in women's imaging, including cardiovascular disorder assessment in pregnant or lactating patients, as well as patients bearing IUDs. Combined efforts between referring clinicians and radiologists are essential for providing the best practice.

When a pregnant patient with an acute problem Is referred to imaging with a specific diagnostic question, it is the radiologist's role to decide whether this question can be answered with a nonionizing modality such as ultrasonography or MR imaging. From the feasibility and/or specific questions asked, it is the radiologist's role to estimate fetal and maternal risk or potential adverse effects of MR imaging and/or IV administration of gadolinium in each case, as well as to structure the examination without compromising diagnostic accuracy. Patient should give informed consent before their procedures.

A careful approach to any MR imaging during pregnancy, including cardiovascular MR imaging with emphasis on minimizing potential acoustic damage and tissue heating, is essential despite primarily theoretic potential fetal damage from the procedure.

Necessary cardiovascular imaging examinations can also be performed in women bearing IUDs, based on the currently available data.

REFERENCES

1. Litmanovich DE, Tack D, Lee KS, et al. Cardiothoracic imaging in the pregnant patient. J Thorac Imaging 2014;29(1):38–49. http://dx.doi.org/10.1097/RTI.0000000000000064.

2. Hartwig V, Giovannetti G, Vanello N, et al. Biological effects and safety in magnetic resonance imaging: a review. Int J Environ Res Public Health 2009;6(6):1778–98. http://dx.doi.org/10.3390/ijerph6061778.

3. Rinck PA. Magnetic resonance in medicine. The basic textbook of the European Magnetic Resonance Forum. 7th edition. 2013. Available at: http://www.magnetic-resonance.org/ch/21-01.html. Accessed September 29, 2014.

4. Kanal E, Barkovich AJ, Bell C, et al. ACR guidance document on MR safe practices: 2013. J Magn Reson Imaging 2013;37(3):501–30. http://dx.doi.org/10.1002/jmri.24011.

5. Shellock FG. Reference manual for magnetic resonance safety, implants and devices. 2014 edition. Playa Del Rey (CA): Biomedical Research Publishing Group; 2014.

6. International Commission on Non-Ionizing Radiation Protection. Amendment to the ICNIRP "Statement on medical magnetic resonance (MR) procedures: protection of patients". Health Phys 2009;97(3):259–61. http://dx.doi.org/10.1097/HP.0b013e3181aff9eb.

7. Schenck JF. Safety of strong, static magnetic fields. J Magn Reson Imaging 2000;12(1):2–19. Available at: http://www.ncbi.nlm.nih.gov/pubmed/10931560. Accessed February 9, 2014.

8. International Commission on Non-Ionizing Radiation Protection. ICNIRP statement on the "Guidelines for limiting exposure to time-varying electric, magnetic, and electromagnetic fields (up to 300 GHz)". Health Phys 2009;97(3):257–8. http://dx.doi.org/10.1097/HP.0b013e3181aff9db.

9. International Commission on Non-Ionizing Radiation Protection. Guidelines on limits of exposure to static magnetic fields. Health Phys 2009;96(4):504–14. http://dx.doi.org/10.1097/01.HP.0000343164.27920.4a.

10. McJury M, Shellock FG. Auditory noise associated with MR procedures: a review. J Magn Reson Imaging 2000;12(1):37–45. Available at: http://www.ncbi.nlm.nih.gov/pubmed/10931563.

11. Shellock FG, Crues JV. MRI bioeffects, safety, and patient management. Los Angeles (CA): Biomedical Research Publishing Group; 2014. p. 720.

12. Ziskin MC, Morrissey J. Thermal thresholds for teratogenicity, reproduction, and development. Int J Hyperthermia 2011;27(4):374–87. http://dx.doi.org/10.3109/02656736.2011.553769.

13. International Electrotechnical Commission (IEC) - Medical electrical equipment - part 2-33: Particular requirements for the basic safety and essential performance of magnetic resonance equipment for medical diagnosis. 2008. Available at: http://www.document-center.com/standards/show/IEC-60601-2-33. Accessed September 29, 2014.

14. ACR manual on contrast media version 9. ACR Committee on drugs and contrast media. 2013. Available at: http://www.acr.org/~/media/ACR/Documents/PDF/QualitySafety/Resources/Contrast%20Manual/2013_Contrast_Media.pdf. Accessed September 29, 2014.

15. Hao D, Ai T, Goerner F, et al. MRI contrast agents: basic chemistry and safety. J Magn Reson Imaging 2012;36(5):1060–71. http://dx.doi.org/10.1002/jmri.23725.

16. Sundgren PC, Leander P. Is administration of gadolinium-based contrast media to pregnant women and small children justified? J Magn Reson Imaging 2011;34(4):750–7. http://dx.doi.org/10.1002/jmri.22413.

17. Wang PI, Chong ST, Kielar AZ, et al. Imaging of pregnant and lactating patients: part 1, evidence-based review and recommendations. AJR Am J Roentgenol 2012;198(4):778–84. http://dx.doi.org/10.2214/AJR.11.7405.

18. Hand JW, Li Y, Hajnal JV. Numerical study of RF exposure and the resulting temperature rise in the foetus during a magnetic resonance procedure. Phys Med Biol 2010;55(4):913–30. http://dx.doi.org/10.1088/0031-9155/55/4/001.

19. De Wilde JP, Rivers AW, Price DL. A review of the current use of magnetic resonance imaging in pregnancy and safety implications for the fetus. Prog Biophys Mol Biol 2005;87(2–3):335–53. http://dx.doi.org/10.1016/j.pbiomolbio.2004.08.010.

20. Graham JM, Edwards MJ. Teratogen update: gestational effects of maternal hyperthermia due to febrile illnesses and resultant patterns of defects in humans. Teratology 1998;58(5):209–21. http://dx.doi.org/10.1002/(SICI)1096-9926(199811)58.

21. Chambers CD. Risks of hyperthermia associated with hot tub or spa use by pregnant women. Birth Defects Res A Clin Mol Teratol 2006;76(8):569–73. http://dx.doi.org/10.1002/bdra.20303.

22. Noise: a hazard for the fetus and newborn. American Academy of Pediatrics. Committee on Environmental Health. Pediatrics 1997;100(4):724–7. Available at: http://www.ncbi.nlm.nih.gov/pubmed/9836852. Accessed February 9, 2014.

23. Webb JA, Thomsen HS. Gadolinium contrast media during pregnancy and lactation. Acta Radiol 2013;54(6):599–600. http://dx.doi.org/10.1177/0284185113484894.

24. Webb JA, Thomsen HS, Morcos SK. The use of iodinated and gadolinium contrast media during pregnancy and lactation. Eur Radiol 2005;15(6):1234–40. http://dx.doi.org/10.1007/s00330-004-2583-y.

25. Normann PT, Joffe P, Martinsen I, et al. Quantification of gadodiamide as Gd in serum, peritoneal dialysate

and faeces by inductively coupled plasma atomic emission spectroscopy and comparative analysis by high-performance liquid chromatography. J Pharm Biomed Anal 2000;22(6):939–47. Available at: http://www.ncbi.nlm.nih.gov/pubmed/10857563.

26. De Santis M, Straface G, Cavaliere AF, et al. Gadolinium periconceptional exposure: pregnancy and neonatal outcome. Acta Obstet Gynecol Scand 2007;86(1):99–101. http://dx.doi.org/10.1080/00016 340600804639.

27. Tremblay E, Thérasse E, Thomassin-Naggara I, et al. Quality initiatives: guidelines for use of medical imaging during pregnancy and lactation. Radiographics 2012;32(3):897–911. http://dx.doi.org/10.1148/rg.323115120.

28. Correia L, Ramos AB, Machado AI, et al. Magnetic resonance imaging and gynecological devices. Contraception 2012;85(6):538–43. http://dx.doi.org/10.1016/j.contraception.2011.10.011.

29. Suh JS, Jeong EK, Shin KH, et al. Minimizing artifacts caused by metallic implants at MR imaging: experimental and clinical studies. AJR Am J Roentgenol 1998;171(5):1207–13. http://dx.doi.org/10.2214/ajr.171.5.9798849.

Arrhythmogenic Right Ventricular Cardiomyopathy/Dysplasia
An Updated Imaging Approach

Stefan L. Zimmerman, MD

KEYWORDS

- Arrhythmogenic right ventricular cardiomyopathy/dysplasia • Task Force Criteria • Cardiac MRI
- Pitfalls

KEY POINTS

- Regional abnormalities of right ventricular (RV) function, such as localized dyskinetic wall motion or microaneurysms, are the hallmark of arrhythmogenic right ventricular cardiomyopathy/dysplasia (ARVC/D).
- Regional wall motion abnormalities and global abnormalities of RV size or function are required to meet major or minor MR imaging Task Force Criteria.
- Although MR imaging can detect fat and fibrosis in the RV wall in ARVC/D patients, neither of these features are part of the diagnostic criteria, in part because of poor reproducibility and lack of specificity.
- Left ventricular abnormalities in ARVC/D are common, with both biventricular and left-dominant forms of the disease increasingly recognized.
- Knowledge of potential pitfalls and mimics in the evaluation of patients suspected of having ARVC/D is important in avoiding misdiagnosis.

INTRODUCTION

Arrhythmogenic right ventricular cardiomyopathy/dysplasia (ARVC/D) is a rare inherited cardiomyopathy characterized by progressive right ventricular (RV) dysfunction caused by fibrofatty replacement of the RV myocardium. Patients have an increased risk of sudden cardiac death from lethal ventricular arrhythmias, which in some cases may be the presenting symptom. Cardiac magnetic resonance (CMR) plays an important role in the diagnostic evaluation of patients and family members suspected of having ARVC/D. This article discusses the epidemiology and pathophysiology of ARVC/D, reviews typical CMR findings and diagnostic criteria, and summarizes potential causes for misdiagnosis in the CMR evaluation of patients suspected of having ARVC/D.

EPIDEMIOLOGY AND PATHOPHYSIOLOGY

ARVC/D is a rare disorder with an estimated prevalence of 1:5000 in the general population.[1] Patients are most often in the second through fifth decade of life with a slight male bias.[2] Patients present with a variety of symptoms ranging from palpitations, syncope, and chest pain to life-threatening arrhythmias. Although rare, ARVC/D

The author has nothing to disclose.

The Russell H. Morgan Department of Radiology and Radiological Sciences, Johns Hopkins University School of Medicine, 601 North Caroline Street, JHOC 3142, Box 0818, Baltimore, MD 21287, USA

E-mail address: stefan.zimmerman@jhmi.edu

Magn Reson Imaging Clin N Am 23 (2015) 69–79
http://dx.doi.org/10.1016/j.mric.2014.09.001
1064-9689/15/$ – see front matter © 2015 Elsevier Inc. All rights reserved.

is an important cause of sudden cardiac death in athletes.[3] Treatment of ARVC/D relies on prevention of sudden death through prophylactic implantation of an internal cardioverter-defibrillator.

ARVC/D is a genetic disorder, although the culprit gene is identified in only approximately 30% to 50% of probands.[4] It is inherited in an autosomal dominant fashion with variable and incomplete penetrance. Five culprit genetic defects have been identified, most of which encode structural proteins crucial in the function of the desmosome, a structure critical to cell-cell junctions. These structural abnormalities result in progressive myocyte death and replacement of the RV myocardium with fat and fibrosis.[5] There is regional variation in the prevalence of ARVC/D-causing mutations; plakophilin-2 (PKP2) is the most common mutation in North American cohorts,[6,7] whereas in some European cohorts, desmoplakin (DSP) and desmoglein (DSG) are more prevalent.[8]

The diagnosis of ARVC/D is challenging for several reasons. Although inherited in an autosomal dominant fashion, ARVC/D has variable penetrance and expressivity. It can present over a wide range of ages with significant differences in phenotypic severity. In one large North American cohort of 108 probands with ARVC/D, age at diagnosis ranged from 12 to 63 years.[7] Screening of family members is particularly challenging, as even if a culprit genetic defect is identified, subjects harboring identical mutations may have dramatic differences in presentations and disease course. Adding to the challenge is the lack of a single specific diagnostic test for ARVC/D. At present, diagnosis is based on a group of clinical, imaging, and histopathologic parameters known as the Task Force Criteria (TFC), which were originally proposed in 1994 and subsequently revised in 2010.[9,10] The TFC designate a group of major and minor criteria, including personal and family history of sudden cardiac death, electrical abnormalities from electrocardiography (ECG) or Holter monitoring, functional and structural abnormalities of the right ventricle from cardiac imaging studies, genetic profile, and RV histopathology. CMR TFC under the 1994 and 2010 proposals are detailed in **Table 1**.

ROLE OF MR IMAGING IN ARRHYTHMOGENIC RIGHT VENTRICULAR CARDIOMYOPATHY/DYSPLASIA

Cardiac MR imaging is uniquely suited for the evaluation of ARVC/D, given its strengths in imaging of the right ventricle. Echocardiography, the first-line noninvasive imaging test for cardiac evaluation, is limited for the right ventricle because of its operator dependency and difficulty resolving the RV wall in the near field. CMR is operator independent and provides high spatial and contrast

---

Table 1
Comparison of original 1994 and revised 2010 CMR Task Force Criteria for the diagnosis of ARVC/D

1994 Task Force Criteria	2010 Task Force Criteria
Major Criteria	
Severe dilatation and reduction of RV EF with no (or only mild) LV impairment	Regional RV akinesia or dyskinesia or dyssynchronous RV contraction
Localized RV aneurysms (akinetic or dyskinetic areas with diastolic bulging)	And 1 of the following:
Severe segmental dilatation of the right ventricle	Ratio of RV end-diastolic volume to BSA $\geq$110 mL/m^2 (male) or $\geq$100 mL/m^2 (female)
	Or RV EF $\leq$40%
Minor Criteria	
Mild global RV dilatation and/or EF reduction with normal left ventricle	Regional RV akinesia or dyskinesia or dyssynchronous RV contraction
Mild segmental dilatation of the right ventricle	And 1 of the following:
Regional RV hypokinesis	Ratio of RV end-diastolic volume to BSA $\geq$100 to <110 mL/m^2 (male) or $\geq$90 to <100 mL/m^2 (female)
	Or RV EF >40% to <45%

Abbreviations: ARVC/D, arrhythmogenic right ventricular cardiomyopathy/dysplasia; BSA, body surface area; EF, ejection fraction; LV, left ventricular; RV, right ventricular.
Adapted from Marcus FI, McKenna WJ, Sherrill D, et al. Diagnosis of arrhythmogenic right ventricular cardiomyopathy/dysplasia: proposed modification of the Task Force Criteria. Eur Heart J 2010;31(7):806–14.

resolution, allowing definitive evaluation of RV function and morphology.[11] Standard CMR ARVC/D protocols typically include cine images for evaluation of cardiac function, dark blood images with and without fat saturation for evaluation of ventricular morphology, and postcontrast late gadolinium enhancement (LGE) images to evaluate for myocardial fibrosis (**Table 2**). As a component of the TFC, MR imaging plays an important role in the diagnostic evaluation of patients with suspected ARVC/D and is frequently crucial to establishment of the diagnosis. As already discussed, ARVC/D is a difficult diagnosis, and patients may present with nonspecific symptoms such as palpitations or chest pain. Electrical abnormalities are common in clinical practice, and the absence of structural disease at MR imaging is important to differentiate ARVC/D from benign abnormalities such as RV outflow tract tachycardia. MR imaging is useful not only for establishing initial diagnosis of ARVC/D but also for screening of family members at risk. Genetic testing is now routinely performed in the management of patients and family members with ARVC/D. As a result, an increasing number of MR imaging examinations will be performed on subjects identified, based not on symptoms but rather on abnormal genetic testing. A recent 2013 study by te Riele and colleagues[6] found that MR imaging may be helpful in this capacity for identifying gene carriers with a high-risk phenotype. In this study, the combination of both MR imaging and electrical abnormalities in ARVC/D gene carriers identified an advanced disease phenotype that was associated with higher risk of subsequent arrhythmic events, whereas none of the subjects with normal MR imaging experienced arrhythmic events at follow-up.

MR IMAGING TASK FORCE CRITERIA

The MR imaging component of the TFC contains 2 elements: (1) qualitative evaluation of regional wall motion and (2) global quantification of RV size and function. Abnormalities in both elements must be present to meet MR imaging criteria. This rule represents an important change from the initial 1994 TFC for which qualitative findings, such as localized aneurysms or segmental RV dilatation, could qualify for major or minor criteria. Quantitative criteria were added with the 2010 revision to limit subjectivity and improve specificity of diagnosis. The effect of these changes was investigated by Vermes and colleagues,[12] who studied 294 patients referred for ARVC/D evaluation, 69 of whom were initially diagnosed with major MR imaging criteria under the 1994 guidelines. After applying 2010 criteria, MR imaging had significantly improved specificity, increasing from 78% by 1994 TFC to 94% with 2010 TFC. However, this came at the expense of reduced sensitivity, with only 4 of 10 patients with ARVC/D meeting major criteria as per 2010 guidelines, compared with 9 of 10 using 1994 criteria. Many fewer subjects met major criteria, and 97% of those previously meeting minor criteria met no criteria at all under 2010 guidelines. Despite these changes to the MR imaging criteria, additional modifications to the clinical portion of the TFC, the most significant of which were changes to ECG criteria, family history criteria, and the inclusion of major criteria points for identification of a

Table 2
Cardiac MR imaging protocol for arrhythmogenic right ventricular cardiomyopathy/dysplasia

	Imaging Sequence		
	T1 Dark Blood	**Bright Blood Cine**	**Delayed Enhancement**
Plane	Axial, SAX	SAX, HLA, RVOT, axial	SAX, Axial
Type	FSE with/without fat suppression	SSFP	Segmented GRE
TR/TE (ms)	1–2/30	2.6/1.3	7.2/3.2
Flip angle (°)	180	40–80	25
Slice thickness (mm)	5	8	8–10
Slice gap (mm)	—	2	2
Field of view (cm)	28–32	36–40	36–10
Inversion time (ms)	—	—	150–250
Temporal resolution (ms)	—	30–40	—

Abbreviations: FSE, fast spin echo; GRE, gradient echo; HLA, horizontal long axis; RVOT, right ventricular outflow tract; SAX, short axis; SSFP, steady-state free precession; TE, echo time; TR, repetition time.

pathogenic ARVC/D-causing mutations, has resulted in an overall increased sensitivity for the diagnosis, particularly among family members of probands.[13]

REGIONAL WALL MOTION ABNORMALITIES

Regional abnormalities of RV wall motion are the characteristic imaging signature of RV dysplasia. These regional abnormalities can manifest as areas of akinesia, dyskinesia, or bulging microaneurysms or macroaneurysms (**Figs. 1** and **2**). Traditionally, ARVC/D in the right ventricle is thought to preferentially involve the RV inflow, outflow, and apical regions, known as the "triangle of dysplasia."[14] This concept was based on early studies in ARVC/D that were biased toward description of subjects with advanced disease. However, a recent study of gene-positive subjects with ARVC/D, many with early identification through family screening, has brought into question this dogma.[15] In this particular study, 74 patients with ARVC/D underwent detailed cardiac MR imaging evaluation to localize wall motion abnormalities. In patients with limited structural disease, regional wall motion abnormalities of the right ventricle were most often found in the inferior wall, the anterolateral wall, and at the interface between these 2 regions, the so-called RV angle (see **Fig. 1**). Involvement of the RV apex was a finding only found in association with advanced structural disease throughout the entire RV. In the same study, these regions corresponded well with low-voltage scar identified by invasive electroanatomic mapping.[15] Cine steady-state free precession bright blood images obtained in axial, short-axis, and RV outflow tract planes are most helpful for identification of these abnormalities. Inferior wall abnormalities in subjects with early disease are best identified on short-axis images; however, care should be taken to distinguish this from dynamic volume averaging of the right atrium resulting from tricuspid annular displacement during the cardiac cycle. For this reason, confirmation of wall motion abnormalities on contiguous slices is recommended. Axial images are particularly helpful for evaluation of the RV outflow tract (see **Fig. 2**).

GLOBAL FUNCTIONAL ABNORMALITIES

Subjects with ARVC/D and structural abnormalities of the right ventricle will most often have reduced RV ejection fraction and RV dilatation. Quantification is typically performed on contiguous short-axis slices covering the right ventricle using dedicated software. Some investigators have proposed the use of either radial or axial cine views through the right ventricle for reduced variability. Quantitative diagnostic thresholds for meeting TFC are provided in **Table 2**. Although CMR is considered the gold standard for RV evaluation, it is not without limitations. Quantification of volumes and function is more challenging for the right ventricle than the left ventricle, given its unusual shape, and interobserver variability for these measures is higher. RV ejection fraction, for instance, demonstrated interobserver coefficients of repeatability (defined as 2 times standard deviation, the least detectable difference when comparing measurements[16]) ranging from 12% to 23% in studies of normal volunteers from experienced imaging centers,[17,18] with end-diastolic volumes varying from 16 to 48 mL.

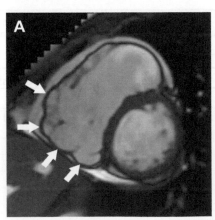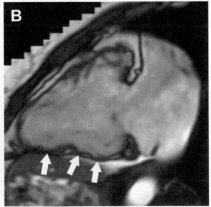

Fig. 1. Short-axis (*A*) and long-axis (*B*) steady-state free precession (SSFP) images obtained from a cardiac MR imaging performed in a 36-year-old woman with Arrhythmogenic right ventricular cardiomyopathy/dysplasia (ARVC/D) meeting MR imaging Task Force Criteria. There are regional wall motion abnormalities manifest as focal areas of outward bulging of the inferior wall, "angle," and anterolateral wall of the right ventricle (*arrows*). The right ventricle is dilated, significantly larger than the left ventricle.

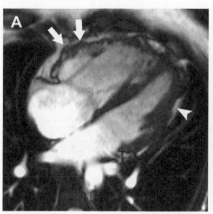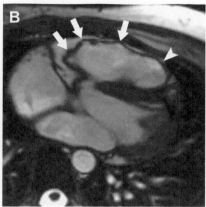

Fig. 2. (*A*) Four-chamber SSFP image obtained during systole in a 29-year-old woman with ARVC/D shows an area of outward bulging in the right ventricular (RV) free wall compatible with regional dyskinesia (*arrows*). Epicardial fat infiltration, with associated etching artifact, involves the apicolateral LV wall (*arrowhead*). (*B*) Axial SSFP image obtained in systole in the region just inferior to the RV outflow tract shows multiple tiny focal bulges, which could be considered microaneurysms (*arrows*). A larger area of dyskinesia is also present, adjacent to the septum (*arrowhead*), which shows outward bulging compared with diastole.

Such differences are important to consider when one realizes that a swing in RV ejection fraction of merely 6%, that is, from 40% to 46%, can change a study from meeting major TFC to none at all (see **Table 1**). Imagers or technologists who perform measurements for these examinations should have adequate training, and in an ideal situation measurements will be made by the same individual to limit variability. Limiting such errors will reduce potential misdiagnosis of ARVC/D.

RIGHT VENTRICULAR FAT

RV fat involvement in ARVC/D is best evaluated with high-resolution spin-echo T1-weighted black blood images obtained with and without fat saturation. On these sequences, fat infiltration is identified by finger-like projections of fat that disrupt the normally smooth interface between epicardial fat and the RV wall (**Fig. 3**).[19] Fat-saturated images may help to confirm the irregularity of the epicardial surface of the right ventricle seen with fat infiltration. In practice, many physicians equate fat identification with the diagnosis of ARVC/D. However, one must bear in mind that the identification of fat in the right ventricle by MR imaging is not part of the current diagnostic criteria, owing to lack of specificity and high interobserver variability. Enthusiasm for the use of MR imaging in this capacity is understood, given that fibrofatty replacement of the right ventricle is the histopathologic hallmark of ARVC/D, and the strengths of MR imaging for tissue characterization. Early reports describing MR imaging characteristics of

patients with ARVC/D fueled this enthusiasm, identifying fat infiltration in a large percentage of patients who met criteria for ARVC/D.[20,21] However, subsequent studies have found that fat assessment with MR imaging in ARVC/D is unreliable. In a 2003 study by Bluemke and colleagues,[22] 13 expert readers evaluated a group of 45 sets of images (7 definite ARVC/D patients, 6 controls, and 32 cases with suspected ARVC/D) and found that fat identification had poor reproducibility; furthermore, there were no differences between groups in prevalence of RV fat. Tandri and colleagues[23] found in 2006 that fat identification lacked reproducibility and specificity compared with regional and global functional abnormalities of the right ventricle. Finally, in the North American Multidisciplinary Study of Right Ventricular Dysplasia published in 2008, RV fat infiltration was identified in only 60% of 42 probands, whereas quantitative estimates of RV function had higher sensitivity and specificity for ARVC/D diagnosis than fat.[24] These reports underscore several challenges to the use of MR fat detection for the diagnosis of ARVC/D. First, limited spatial resolution in MR imaging makes it difficult to distinguish fat infiltration within the thin RV free wall from adjacent epicardial fat.[19] Even when correctly identified, RV fat infiltration is not uncommonly found in the RV free wall and RV outflow tract in patients with no history of cardiac disease, and seems to increase with aging.[25] In autopsy studies, fat in the right ventricle is a frequent finding, with adipocytes in the wall interspersed with myocytes. Unlike ARVC/D, however, the RV wall becomes thickened and there is no

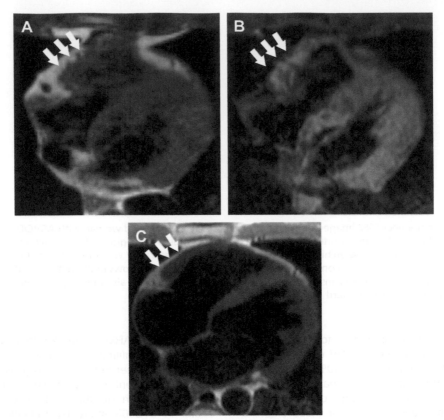

Fig. 3. (*A*) Axial double-inversion recovery dark blood image obtained in a 51-year-old man with ARVC/D shows the typical finger-like infiltration of fat from the epicardial surface of the RV wall in the basilar free wall (*arrows*). (*B*) On fat-saturated images, irregularity of the epicardial surface of the RV wall caused by fat infiltration is well demonstrated (*arrows*). (*C*) Normal RV wall on an axial dark blood image for comparison. There is a smooth epicardial contour, with the interface between epicardial fat and the RV wall clearly defined (*arrows*).

associated fibrosis (**Fig. 4**).[25,26] Of note, only subjects with ARVC/D will demonstrate wall motion abnormalities in association with fat infiltration, which may help differentiate pathologic fat in ARVC/D from fat infiltration related to aging or other causes.[27]

RIGHT VENTRICULAR LATE GADOLINIUM ENHANCEMENT

ARVC/D is characterized by both fibrosis and fat in the right ventricle, so it is not surprising that LGE is frequently identified in the right ventricle of these patients. LGE is typically identified as regional high signal in the RV free wall and trabeculations, and often corresponds to regional dysfunction on cine images (**Fig. 5**). In a study by Tandri and colleagues,[28] 30 patients were evaluated with MR imaging for suspected ARVC/D. Of these, 8 of 12 (67%) who met ARVC/D diagnostic criteria had LGE in the right ventricle on MR imaging, compared with none of 18 patients who did not meet criteria. In those patients with prior

biopsy, LGE correlated well with identification of fibrofatty infiltration at histopathology. Identification of LGE in the right ventricle also correlated with increased risk of induced sustained ventricular tachycardia. Fibrosis is the anatomic substrate for arrhythmia and, as such, LGE MR imaging has the potential to map arrhythmogenic regions in the right ventricle to target for ablation procedures. Two previous studies have investigated combining invasive electroanatomic (EAM) voltage mapping data with LGE MR imaging findings. Santangeli and colleagues[29] found in 2010 that LGE at MR imaging correlated closely with low-voltage areas, but underperformed in comparison with EAM, with LGE absent in 5 of 13 patients with low-voltage scar by EAM. Marra and colleagues[30] presented similar results in 2012; although LGE at MR imaging correlated well with low-voltage areas by EAM, MR imaging lacked sensitivity, with many more scars identified on EAM than were visualized by MR imaging. Taken together, these results indicate that LGE has promise for identification of RV scar in ARVC for arrhythmia risk stratification

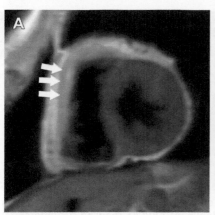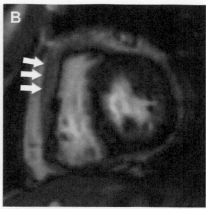

Fig. 4. Age-related fat infiltration in a 44-year-old woman with no history of ARVC/D. (*A*) Short-axis double-inversion recovery dark blood image showing high signal intensity in a thickened RV wall caused by diffuse fat infiltration (*arrows*). The dark line adjacent to the arrows represents the interface between RV wall and epicardial fat adjacent to the right ventricle. (*B*) Similar findings are seen on short-axis SSFP images (*arrows*); there was no regional wall motion abnormality on cine images.

or ablation planning, but improvements in spatial and contrast resolution will be needed for greater sensitivity.

THE LEFT VENTRICLE IN ARRHYTHMOGENIC RIGHT VENTRICULAR CARDIOMYOPATHY/ DYSPLASIA

Left ventricular (LV) abnormalities are not uncommon in ARVC/D patients. The prevalence and

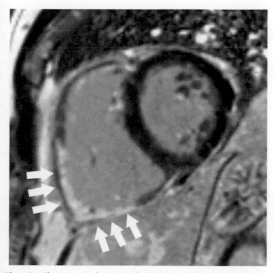

Fig. 5. Short-axis late gadolinium enhancement image obtained in a 56-year-old man with ARVC/D shows segmentally increased signal intensity in the inferior and anterolateral walls of the right ventricle (*arrows*), which corresponded to a regional wall motion abnormality on cine images.

severity of LV abnormalities relative to RV involvement is likely related to genotype,[31] and varies depending on the patient cohort, from greater than 80% in a large group of probands and relatives from the United Kingdom[8] to 38% from a recently described cohort of gene-positive North American and Dutch subjects with ARVC/D.[15] Three patterns of LV involvement in ARVC/D have been described.[8] The classic ARVC/D pattern has isolated RV disease without LV abnormalities. This pattern is more often found in North American cohorts, in which the PKP2 mutation is most common.[7,32,33] The biventricular pattern shows involvement of both ventricles, usually characterized by regional RV dysfunction, subepicardial fatty infiltration in apicolateral and inferobasal wall of the left ventricle, and preserved LV function (see **Fig. 2**).[32,34] In the left-dominant pattern, LV manifestations of the disease predominate with relatively mild RV abnormalities. This pattern of disease has been found more frequently in cohorts from the United Kingdom, where desmoplakin mutations are more common.[35] Subjects demonstrate regional LV dysfunction, mid-wall or subepicardial LV LGE, and a higher frequency of ventricular tachyarrhythmias (**Fig. 6**). This pattern is likely underrecognized and is often misdiagnosed as sarcoidosis or myocarditis, likely because of a lack of specific criteria for diagnosis.[35] It is clear that the pathologic desmosomal mutations responsible for ARVC/D can affect either ventricle, and some have suggested renaming the disease "arrhythmogenic cardiomyopathy."[36] Other investigators have called for inclusion of LV abnormalities in future TFC modifications.[35]

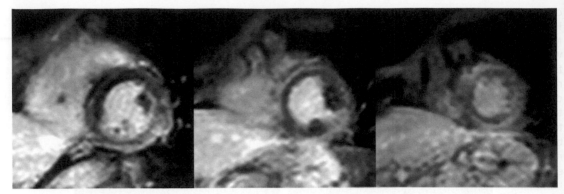

Fig. 6. Short-axis late gadolinium enhancement images obtained at the base, mid-cavity, and apex (*left to right*) in a 56-year-old man diagnosed with left ventricle–predominant ARVC/D, showing circumferential mid-wall late enhancement throughout the left ventricle, typical for left-dominant ARVC/D. ARVC/D Task Force Criteria were met based on family history of ARVC/D and the presence of additional RV structural abnormalities.

CHALLENGES IN EVALUATION OF ARRHYTHMOGENIC RIGHT VENTRICULAR CARDIOMYOPATHY/DYSPLASIA

MR imaging evaluation of ARVC/D is challenging for several reasons. Referrals to MR imaging centers for ARVC/D are common; however, owing to the rarity of the disease, most imagers may never encounter a real case of ARVC/D outside of static images from journal articles and textbooks. Normal variants of RV wall motion and various mimics can be mistaken for ARVC/D at MR imaging. Right ventricular wall motion is more complex than that on the left side, and contraction patterns are variable even among normal subjects. Subjective bulging of the free wall on axial cine images is common, found in 63% to 86% of normal patients on cine images in the axial plane.[37,38] These bulges are most often found around the moderator band insertion into the apicolateral free wall of the right ventricle, and are less commonly seen in the short-axis and horizontal long-axis planes (**Fig. 7**).[37] For these reasons, wall motion abnormalities should be routinely confirmed in more than 1 imaging plane and contiguous slices. Distinction of findings that are within the normal range of RV wall motion from pathologic abnormalities characteristic of ARVC/D requires considerable reader experience that is often limited to referral centers. Inexperienced readers may be more likely to attribute these normal variants to ARVC/D, given the potentially grave implications of a missed diagnosis. In addition, inappropriate weight is often assigned to non-TFC findings such as fat and late gadolinium enhancement in the RV wall, which were not included in the TFC because of concerns over subjectivity and lack of specificity.[10] In a study by Bomma and colleagues[39] in 2004, 65 MR

imaging examinations from subjects referred to a tertiary care center for a second opinion regarding the diagnosis of ARVC/D were reviewed. Among the MR imaging examinations, 92% were read as abnormal by the referring center, and most abnormalities (71%) were the qualitative presence of RV intramyocardial fat and/or wall thinning. On secondary review by expert readers, none of these qualitative findings were confirmed.

Several pathologic conditions can mimic ARVC/D at MR imaging. The most common of these is displacement of the right ventricle from pectus excavatum or scoliosis.[40] In these patients, the normal RV shape is distorted with relative basilar

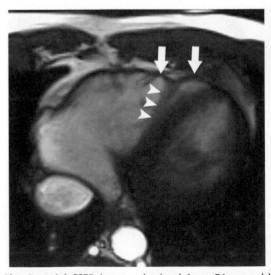

Fig. 7. Axial SSFP image obtained in a 51-year-old man being evaluated for ARVC/D shows apicolateral bulging (*arrows*) caused by insertion of the moderator band (*arrowheads*) on the free wall of the right ventricle, a normal variant of RV wall motion that should not be mistaken for pathology.

compression and apical enlargement (**Fig. 8**). However, in a review of 18 patients in whom MR imaging findings found pectus deformity, RV wall motion abnormalities, diminished RV systolic function, or RV dilatation, none of the patients met ARVC/D diagnostic criteria.[41] Other mimics of ARVC/D include RV volume overload secondary to occult left to right shunts and RV LGE related to myocarditis or sarcoidosis. A previous study by Steckman and colleagues[42] demonstrated significant overlap between patients with cardiac sarcoidosis and ARVC/D. Both subsets of patients demonstrated RV enlargement and reduced RV function, but patients with sarcoidosis had more extensive delayed enhancement and more frequent LV involvement than ARVC/D patients.

Physiologic enlargement of the right ventricle that occurs in highly conditioned athletes can also mimic ARVC/D. A study by Luijkx and colleagues[43] in 2012 showed that 86% of male healthy athletes and 80% of female athletes met volume thresholds for ARVC/D diagnostic criteria. Of importance, none of these patients demonstrated regional wall motion abnormalities that would be necessary to meet major or minor criteria. These findings and those in subjects with RV displacement emphasize the importance of combination of qualitative and quantitative findings to avoid misdiagnosis, and further reinforce the need for global evaluation of all criteria rather than overreliance on MR imaging.

SUMMARY

MR imaging plays a crucial role in evaluation of patients with suspected ARVC/D given its unparalleled assessment of RV structure and function. However, these strengths must be balanced against several challenges to reliable assessment of ARVC/D. The most notable of these are subjectivity in assessment of RV wall motion, variability in quantification of RV size and function, overlap of MR imaging criteria with physiologic and pathologic processes that affect the right ventricle, such as athlete's heart, cardiac displacement, and sarcoidosis, and overreliance on morphologic abnormalities such as RV fat infiltration. Knowledge of these potential errors and adherence to the 2010 TFC will help imagers avoid misdiagnosis.

ACKNOWLEDGEMENTS

I would like to thank the exceptional group of physicians, geneticists, and research fellows of the Johns Hopkins ARVD/C program.

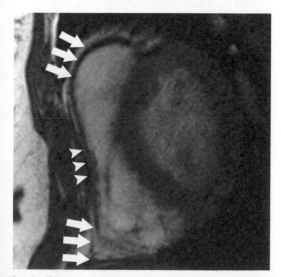

Fig. 8. Short-axis SSFP image obtained in a 61-year-old woman with pectus deformity misdiagnosed with ARVC/D at initial evaluation due to identification of focal wall motion abnormalities at MR imaging. The pectus deformity results in constriction of the mid-portion of the right ventricle (*arrowheads*) and the relative increase in size of the RV outflow tract and inferior portions of the right ventricle (*arrows*), which was misinterpreted as a wall motion abnormality. On cine images, contraction of the right ventricle was normal.

REFERENCES

1. Romero J, Mejia-Lopez E, Manrique C, et al. Arrhythmogenic right ventricular cardiomyopathy (ARVC/D): a systematic literature review. Clin Med Insights Cardiol 2013;7:97–114.
2. Dalal D, Nasir K, Bomma C, et al. Arrhythmogenic right ventricular dysplasia: a United States experience. Circulation 2005;112(25):3823–32.
3. Thiene G, Nava A, Corrado D, et al. Right ventricular cardiomyopathy and sudden death in young people. N Engl J Med 1988;318(3):129–33.
4. Marcus FI, Edson S, Towbin JA. Genetics of arrhythmogenic right ventricular cardiomyopathy: a practical guide for physicians. J Am Coll Cardiol 2013; 61(19):1945–8.
5. Saffitz JE. The pathobiology of arrhythmogenic cardiomyopathy. Annu Rev Pathol 2011;6:299–321.
6. te Riele AS, Bhonsale A, James CA, et al. Incremental value of cardiac magnetic resonance imaging in arrhythmic risk stratification of arrhythmogenic right ventricular dysplasia/cardiomyopathy-associated desmosomal mutation carriers. J Am Coll Cardiol 2013;62(19):1761–9.
7. Marcus FI, Zareba W, Calkins H, et al. Arrhythmogenic right ventricular cardiomyopathy/dysplasia clinical presentation and diagnostic evaluation: results from the North American Multidisciplinary Study. Heart Rhythm 2009;6(7):984–92.

8. Sen-Chowdhry S, Syrris P, Ward D, et al. Clinical and genetic characterization of families with arrhythmogenic right ventricular dysplasia/cardiomyopathy provides novel insights into patterns of disease expression. Circulation 2007;115(13):1710–20.

9. McKenna WJ, Thiene G, Nava A, et al. Diagnosis of arrhythmogenic right ventricular dysplasia/cardiomyopathy. Task Force of the Working Group Myocardial and Pericardial Disease of the European Society of Cardiology and of the Scientific Council on Cardiomyopathies of the International Society and Federation of Cardiology. Br Heart J 1994;71(3):215–8.

10. Marcus FI, McKenna WJ, Sherrill D, et al. Diagnosis of arrhythmogenic right ventricular cardiomyopathy/dysplasia: proposed modification of the Task Force Criteria. Eur Heart J 2010;31(7):806–14.

11. Hundley WG, Bluemke DA, Finn JP, et al. ACCF/ACR/AHA/NASCI/SCMR 2010 expert consensus document on cardiovascular magnetic resonance: a report of the American College of Cardiology Foundation Task Force on Expert Consensus Documents. J Am Coll Cardiol 2010;55(23):2614–62.

12. Vermes E, Strohm O, Otmani A, et al. Impact of the revision of arrhythmogenic right ventricular cardiomyopathy/dysplasia task force criteria on its prevalence by CMR criteria. JACC Cardiovasc Imaging 2011;4(3):282–7.

13. Cox MG, van der Smagt JJ, Noorman M, et al. Arrhythmogenic right ventricular dysplasia/cardiomyopathy diagnostic task force criteria: impact of new task force criteria. Circ Arrhythm Electrophysiol 2010;3(2):126–33.

14. Marcus FI, Fontaine GH, Guiraudon G, et al. Right ventricular dysplasia: a report of 24 adult cases. Circulation 1982;65(2):384–98.

15. Te Riele AS, James CA, Philips B, et al. Mutation-positive arrhythmogenic right ventricular dysplasia/cardiomyopathy: the triangle of dysplasia displaced. J Cardiovasc Electrophysiol 2013;24(12):1311–20.

16. Sardanelli F. Biostatistics for radiologists: planning, performing, writing a radiological study. New York: Springer; 2008.

17. Alfakih K, Plein S, Thiele H, et al. Normal human left and right ventricular dimensions for MRI as assessed by turbo gradient echo and steady-state free precession imaging sequences. J Magn Reson Imaging 2003;17(3):323–9.

18. Teo KS, Carbone A, Piantadosi C, et al. Cardiac MRI assessment of left and right ventricular parameters in healthy Australian normal volunteers. Heart Lung Circ 2008;17(4):313–7.

19. Castillo E, Tandri H, Rodriguez ER, et al. Arrhythmogenic right ventricular dysplasia: ex vivo and in vivo fat detection with black-blood MR imaging. Radiology 2004;232(1):38–48.

20. Tandri H, Calkins H, Nasir K, et al. Magnetic resonance imaging findings in patients meeting task force criteria for arrhythmogenic right ventricular dysplasia. J Cardiovasc Electrophysiol 2003;14(5):476–82.

21. Auffermann W, Wichter T, Breithardt G, et al. Arrhythmogenic right ventricular disease: MR imaging versus angiography. AJR Am J Roentgenol 1993;161(3):549–55.

22. Bluemke DA, Krupinski EA, Ovitt T, et al. MR Imaging of arrhythmogenic right ventricular cardiomyopathy: morphologic findings and interobserver reliability. Cardiology 2003;99(3):153–62.

23. Tandri H, Castillo E, Ferrari VA, et al. Magnetic resonance imaging of arrhythmogenic right ventricular dysplasia: sensitivity, specificity, and observer variability of fat detection versus functional analysis of the right ventricle. J Am Coll Cardiol 2006;48(11):2277–84.

24. Tandri H, Macedo R, Calkins H, et al. Role of magnetic resonance imaging in arrhythmogenic right ventricular dysplasia: insights from the North American arrhythmogenic right ventricular dysplasia (ARVD/C) study. Am Heart J 2008;155(1):147–53.

25. Kimura F, Matsuo Y, Nakajima T, et al. Myocardial fat at cardiac imaging: how can we differentiate pathologic from physiologic fatty infiltration? Radiographics 2010;30(6):1587–602.

26. Burke AP, Farb A, Tashko G, et al. Arrhythmogenic right ventricular cardiomyopathy and fatty replacement of the right ventricular myocardium: are they different diseases? Circulation 1998;97(16):1571–80.

27. Macedo R, Prakasa K, Tichnell C, et al. Marked lipomatous infiltration of the right ventricle: MRI findings in relation to arrhythmogenic right ventricular dysplasia. AJR Am J Roentgenol 2007;188(5):W423–7.

28. Tandri H, Saranathan M, Rodriguez ER, et al. Noninvasive detection of myocardial fibrosis in arrhythmogenic right ventricular cardiomyopathy using delayed-enhancement magnetic resonance imaging. J Am Coll Cardiol 2005;45(1):98–103.

29. Santangeli P, Pieroni M, Dello Russo A, et al. Noninvasive diagnosis of electroanatomic abnormalities in arrhythmogenic right ventricular cardiomyopathy. Circ Arrhythm Electrophysiol 2010;3(6):632–8.

30. Marra MP, Leoni L, Bauce B, et al. Imaging study of ventricular scar in arrhythmogenic right ventricular cardiomyopathy: comparison of 3D standard electroanatomical voltage mapping and contrast-enhanced cardiac magnetic resonance. Circ Arrhythm Electrophysiol 2012;5(1):91–100.

31. Te Riele AS, Bhonsale A, Burt JR, et al. Genotype-specific pattern of LV involvement in ARVD/C. JACC Cardiovasc Imaging 2012;5(8):849–51.

32. Dalal D, Tandri H, Judge DP, et al. Morphologic variants of familial arrhythmogenic right ventricular

dysplasia/cardiomyopathy a genetics-magnetic resonance imaging correlation study. J Am Coll Cardiol 2009;53(15):1289–99.

33. Dalal D, Molin LH, Piccini J, et al. Clinical features of arrhythmogenic right ventricular dysplasia/cardiomyopathy associated with mutations in plakophilin-2. Circulation 2006;113(13):1641–9.

34. Corrado D, Basso C, Thiene G, et al. Spectrum of clinicopathologic manifestations of arrhythmogenic right ventricular cardiomyopathy/dysplasia: a multicenter study. J Am Coll Cardiol 1997;30(6): 1512–20.

35. Sen-Chowdhry S, Syrris P, Prasad SK, et al. Left-dominant arrhythmogenic cardiomyopathy: an underrecognized clinical entity. J Am Coll Cardiol 2008; 52(25):2175–87.

36. Basso C, Corrado D, Thiene G. Arrhythmogenic right ventricular cardiomyopathy: what's in a name? From a congenital defect (dysplasia) to a genetically determined cardiomyopathy (dystrophy). Am J Cardiol 2010;106(2):275–7.

37. Sievers B, Addo M, Franken U, et al. Right ventricular wall motion abnormalities found in healthy subjects by cardiovascular magnetic resonance imaging and characterized with a new segmental model. J Cardiovasc Magn Reson 2004;6(3):601–8.

38. Fritz J, Solaiyappan M, Tandri H, et al. Right ventricle shape and contraction patterns and relation to magnetic resonance imaging findings. J Comput Assist Tomogr 2005;29(6):725–33.

39. Bomma C, Rutberg J, Tandri H, et al. Misdiagnosis of arrhythmogenic right ventricular dysplasia/cardiomyopathy. J Cardiovasc Electrophysiol 2004;15(3): 300–6.

40. Quarta G, Husain SI, Flett AS, et al. Arrhythmogenic right ventricular cardiomyopathy mimics: role of cardiovascular magnetic resonance. J Cardiovasc Magn Reson 2013;15:16.

41. Oezcan S, Attenhofer Jost CH, Pfyffer M, et al. Pectus excavatum: echocardiography and cardiac MRI reveal frequent pericardial effusion and right-sided heart anomalies. Eur Heart J Cardiovasc Imaging 2012;13(8):673–9.

42. Steckman DA, Schneider PM, Schuller JL, et al. Utility of cardiac magnetic resonance imaging to differentiate cardiac sarcoidosis from arrhythmogenic right ventricular cardiomyopathy. Am J Cardiol 2012;110(4):575–9.

43. Luijkx T, Velthuis BK, Prakken NH, et al. Impact of revised Task Force Criteria: distinguishing the athlete's heart from ARVC/D using cardiac magnetic resonance imaging. Eur J Prev Cardiol 2012;19(4):885–91.

MR Imaging Evaluation of Pericardial Constriction

Robert Groves, MD[a], Danielle Chan, MD[b], Marianna Zagurovskaya, MD[a], Shawn D. Teague, MD[b],*

KEYWORDS

- Pericardial constriction • Constrictive pericarditis • Cardiac MR imaging

KEY POINTS

- The pericardium is an important component of the heart, with both anatomic and physiologic roles that are critical to ensuring normal cardiac function.
- Pericardial constriction has many causes and is often a source of significant morbidity and mortality.
- Cardiac MR imaging provides clinicians with comprehensive information, both about the pericardium and its effect on cardiac function, in addition to ancillary findings that may be missed by other modalities.
- Multiple other imaging techniques, such as computed tomography, echocardiography, and cardiac catheterization, are often used with clinical findings to provide a confident diagnosis.
- Accurate diagnosis of pericardial constriction and differentiation from restrictive cardiomyopathy are vital to provide prompt and appropriate treatment.

INTRODUCTION

The pericardium is a component of the heart with multiple anatomic and physiologic roles critical to ensuring normal cardiac function. One of its major roles is acting as a barrier to inflammatory disease, which constitutes a spectrum from acute pericarditis to chronic constriction.[1] Some additional roles include maintaining normal heart positioning within the chest, limiting acute myocardial distention, and enhancing the normal interaction of the ventricles. These roles make the pericardium, both its anatomic and physiologic properties, a vital part of normal heart health.

Comprehensive evaluation[2] of both the pericardium and the heart as a whole is an invaluable tool for clinicians faced with treating pericardial constriction and differentiating it from a restrictive cardiomyopathy, which can have a similar presentation but a different management strategy.

CAUSES

Pericardial constriction is commonly an idiopathic phenomenon.[3,4] The 2 most common known causes of pericardial constriction in the developed world are prior cardiac surgery (18%), particularly coronary artery bypass grafting, and radiation therapy (13%), especially when the mediastinum is directly within the treatment field.[3] In the past, infection (particularly tuberculosis) was the most common cause and remains the most common cause in developing countries and immunosuppressed patients. Overall, infectious pericarditis of all types, including both viral and fungal organisms, accounts for up to 16% of cases according to some estimates.[3]

ANATOMY/PHYSIOLOGY

The pericardium is inelastic and made up of 2 layers: the visceral pericardium (which is adherent

Disclosure: The authors have nothing to disclose.
[a] Department of Radiology, Virginia Commonwealth University, 1250 E Marshall St, Richmond, VA 23219, USA;
[b] Department of Radiology, Indiana University, 550 North University Boulevard, Room 0663, Indianapolis, IN 46202, USA
* Corresponding author.
E-mail address: sdteague@iupui.edu

Magn Reson Imaging Clin N Am 23 (2015) 81–87
http://dx.doi.org/10.1016/j.mric.2014.09.003
1064-9689/15/$ – see front matter © 2015 Elsevier Inc. All rights reserved.

to the epicardium) and the more fibrous parietal layer. These layers are separated by a potential space that can normally contain up to 50 mL of fluid. This potential space is tolerant of slow filling with fluid, explaining why large effusions (>50 mL) often do not have immediate deleterious effects on cardiac motion or result in cardiac tamponade. The pericardium surrounds the heart and also encases portions of the great vessels with normal attachments to both the sternum and diaphragm.[2] The pericardium is normally 2 to 3 mm thick, as seen in **Figs. 1** and **2**. Abnormal thickening is defined as greater than 4 mm.[2] Pericardial constriction is defined as abnormal thickening and adhesion of the pericardial layers that limits normal ventricular distention and results in impaired ventricular filling. On histology, this thickening represents fibrosis and scarring.[5] The abnormal thickening may be seen diffusely throughout the pericardium, or focally, frequently along the right ventricular free wall.

When the pericardium becomes thickened and noncompliant the result is uniformly increased filling pressures in all cardiac chambers. For example, increased filling pressure in the left atrium results in rapid left ventricular filling, particularly in early diastole. Overall stroke volumes throughout the heart are decreased, primarily because of reduced preload. There is also increased ventricular interdependence through septal interactions, which results in the characteristic septal bounce on imaging, as detailed later. In addition, normal respiratory transmission of intrathoracic pressure changes to the cardiac chambers is lost. However, contractility is preserved. Therefore, there is an exaggerated respiratory variation in both inflow velocity and ventricular filling in patients with constrictive pericarditis.

MR Imaging Evaluation

MR imaging has become the gold standard for the complete evaluation of the pericardium and the physiologic effects of pericardial constriction. A typical protocol is detailed in **Table 1**. Advantages include the noninvasive technique, lack of ionizing radiation, and providing detailed physiologic information regarding cardiac function and wall motion in addition to anatomic evaluation of the pericardium. The high temporal/spatial resolution and exceptional soft tissue differentiation provide an excellent evaluation of the pericardium. Disadvantages include cost as well as being a more technically difficult examination to perform: both for the patient because of numerous breath holds and long acquisition time relative to computed tomography (CT), and also for the technologist and/or physician performing the study because of the complexity of cardiac MR imaging. One significant disadvantage is the poor ability of MR imaging with respect to detecting even large amounts of calcification. However, this limitation may be negligible, because many cases of constriction have no calcification present.

Signs of pericardial constriction on MR imaging

On MR imaging, the normal pericardium should be less than 4 mm in thickness. It is typically intermediate in signal intensity on both T1-weighted and T2-weighted imaging but is accentuated by the adjacent high signal fat on most sequences. Multiplanar evaluation with MR imaging allows the detection of more subtle focal areas of thickening that may be missed on other modalities. In constrictive pericarditis, thickening may be focal or diffuse. When focal, the right heart border is frequently involved. **Fig. 3** shows a globally

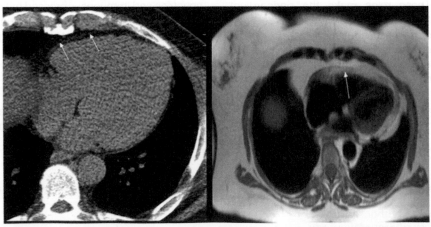

Fig. 1. (*Left*) Axial noncontrast computed tomography image shows a normal pericardial thickness (*arrows*). (*Right*) Axial double inversion recovery image shows a normal pericardial thickness (*arrow*).

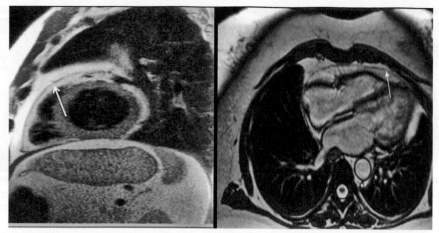

Fig. 2. MR dark blood short-axis (*left*) and bright blood 4-chamber (*right*) views show the normal appearance of the myocardium (*arrows*). Short-axis views can be particularly valuable for evaluation of the right ventricular free wall pericardium, which is a common location for focal thickening.

Table 1
Typical MR imaging protocol for evaluation of the pericardium

Sequence	Plane	Details	Value
3-plane localizer scouts	Axial, coronal, sagittal	5–7 s	Localization of pertinent anatomy
DIR-FSE (black blood) SSFP (bright blood)	Axial, sagittal	8-mm slices through the chest; no gap	Anatomic overview
Cine SSFP	SA, 4Ch, 2Ch	Base to apex, high TR 2–4 slices centrally 1–2 slices centrally	Evaluate wall motion, ventricular function
Real-time images	SA, 4Ch	1–2 min each; may image at multiple levels No breath hold	Evaluate interventricular septal motion Evaluate myocardial-pericardial tethering
Myocardial tagging	SA, 4Ch	10-s to 15-s acquisition Approx 1-cm line gap Approx 45° angle (to the transverse plane)	Evaluate myocardial-pericardial tethering
Immediate postcontrast	SA, 2Ch, 4Ch	10–15 s each; 2–6 slices Approx 1–2 min after injection	Evaluate for acute inflammation
TI scout Delayed post contrast	SA 1 slice midventricle SA, 2Ch, 4Ch	Select inversion time to maximally null myocardium (typically around 300 ms) Single-shot SSFP bright blood Approx 8–10 min after injection	Optimal myocardial nulling to accentuate abnormal enhancement Evaluate for chronic inflammation, fibrosis, masses

High-TR images obtained with at least 30 phases per cardiac cycle.
Contrast medium is gadolinium based, dosed by weight (typically 15–30 mL for an adult).
Abbreviations: 2Ch, 2 chamber; 4Ch, 4 chamber; DIR-FSE, double inversion recovery fast spin echo; SA, short axis; SSFP, steady state free precession; TI, time to inversion; TR, temporal resolution.

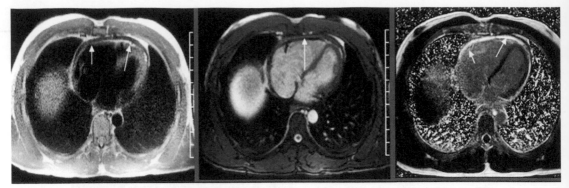

Fig. 3. Four-chamber MR dark blood (*left*), bright blood (*center*), and a novel dark blood postcontrast image (*right*) show abnormal pericardial thickening and global abnormal delayed pericardial enhancement (*arrows*).

thickened pericardium. Although it is frequently seen, there is some evidence to suggest that thickening is not necessarily present.[6]

Another feature of constrictive pericarditis is abnormal tubular morphology of the ventricles as well as biatrial enlargement, as seen in **Fig. 4**. This abnormal morphology is the result of pressure changes in the cardiac chambers related to the abnormal inelasticity of the fibrotic pericardium.

Abnormal motion of the interventricular septum during early diastole, the so-called septal bounce, is another common imaging finding in pericardial constriction. The septum initially moves toward and then away from the left ventricle, a finding that is often accentuated in deep inspiration, as seen in real-time imaging. Reduced ventricular compliance from increasing pressure results in abnormal ventricular interdependence (ie, increasing volume in one ventricle leads to a decreased volume in the other ventricle).[7] This sign is highly specific for constrictive pericarditis[8] and is shown in **Fig. 5**.

Other noncardiac signs of constriction include dilatation of the inferior vena cava with resultant hepatic venous congestion (**Fig. 6**). Ascites and pleural effusions are other indirect findings that can occur but are nonspecific.

MR imaging technique

A typical protocol for the evaluation of pericardial constriction can be seen in **Table 1**. A typical study takes approximately 30 to 40 minutes of scan time.

Pericardial thickening can be measured in various planes and pulse sequences. Double inversion recovery fast spin echo (DIR-FSE) images in the axial or 4-chamber views are typically very accurate at delineating the pericardium, facilitating measurements of its thickness. Cine steady state free precession (SSFP) images in both 4-chamber and short-axis views are also valuable for additional assessment of regional tethering caused by adhesions. Normal pericardium does not enhance after the administration of intravenous contrast media; thus, postcontrast images showing pericardial enhancement suggest that significant inflammation is likely present (**Fig. 7**). Images may be obtained immediately and/or after a 10-minute delay. Immediate enhancement suggests active/acute inflammation.

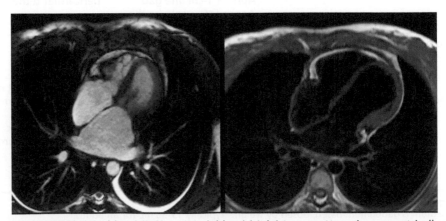

Fig. 4. Four-chamber MR bright blood (*left*) and dark blood (*right*) images. Note the symmetrically dilated atria and abnormal tubular morphology of the heart. Pericardial thickening is also present.

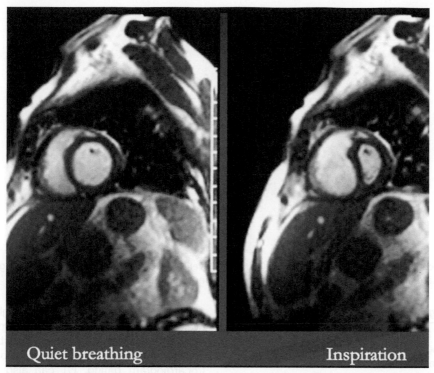

Quiet breathing | Inspiration

Fig. 5. Cine steady state free precession short-axis images show accentuated abnormal septal motion with deep inspiration.

Myocardial tagging (**Fig. 8**) can be performed in multiple planes, most commonly in the 4-chamber plane, which is optimal for evaluation of the pericardium along the right ventricular free wall. Tag lines are seen as dark saturation bands 4 to 5 mm thick

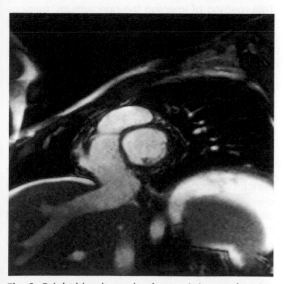

Fig. 6. Bright blood pseudo–short-axis image showing sequelae of pericardial constriction. Note the markedly dilated inferior vena cava and hepatic veins. A pleural effusion is also present.

and typically spaced at intervals of approximately 1 cm over the entire image. In normal patients, these bands break (lose continuity) at the parietal and visceral pericardium during the cardiac cycle, which indicates a normal sliding motion between the pericardial layers. In patients with pericardial constriction and adhesions between these layers, the bands bend but remain unbroken, indicating abnormal tethering of the pericardium.[9]

Cine SSFP short-axis images can be performed with high temporal resolution (approximately 30 phases per cardiac cycle), allowing the detailed evaluation of the pathognomonic abnormal motion of the interventricular septum. However, these images do not take advantage of the accentuated abnormal septal motion during inspiration, because they are acquired over multiple heartbeats and typically during a breath hold. Real-time cine images, typically in the short-axis or 4-chamber views, are acquired without breath hold during the respiratory cycle. This lack of breath hold can be especially helpful in subtle cases of abnormal septal motion, which is typically accentuated during inspiration. The imaging finding of abnormal septal motion is also valuable in distinguishing constriction from restrictive cardiomyopathy, which is commonly in the differential diagnosis and requires a different treatment strategy.

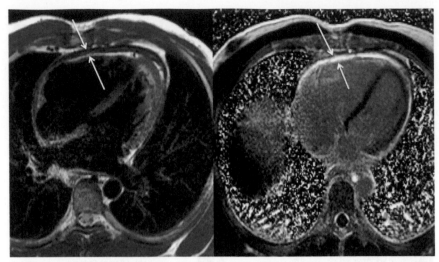

Fig. 7. Four-chamber black blood precontrast (*left*) and novel black blood postcontrast (*right*) images. Note the diffuse pericardial thickening and abnormal delayed enhancement (*arrows*).

Other Imaging Techniques

Computed tomography

The major advantage of CT compared with MR imaging in the evaluation of the pericardium is the detection of calcifications, as shown in **Fig. 9**. Even very small amounts of calcification are easily identified on CT. The thickness of the pericardium can also be accurately assessed, as can the presence or absence of pericardial fluid. Additional information that can be gained with the proper use of CT includes evaluation of the coronary arteries, including anatomy and the presence or absence

of coronary atherosclerosis, although complete evaluation of these vascular structures requires iodinated contrast media, which may be contraindicated in some patients. With retrospective electrocardiogram gating, CT can also provide an estimate of left ventricular function and wall motion, although this requires a much higher dose of radiation compared with the nonionizing MR imaging. In addition, the temporal resolution of CT is lower than that of MR imaging and subsequently may not detect more subtle wall motion abnormalities, particularly septal bounce.

Echocardiography

This method of imaging the pericardium, particularly transesophageal echo, can evaluate several of the findings that suggest pericardial constriction, including pericardial thickening and abnormal septal bounce during diastole.[7] However, evaluation with a transesophageal approach is more invasive than MR imaging and requires sedation, which is typically not necessary for MR imaging. Doppler flow velocities, particularly the mitral and tricuspid inflow velocities, can have a characteristic variation in the presence of diseased pericardium, which has good sensitivity and specificity for pericardial constriction, although there is some overlap with pericardial tamponade.[10] In both constriction and pericardial tamponade, mitral inflow velocity decreases after inspiration and increases after expiration. Tricuspid inflow velocity has the opposite pattern, increasing after inspiration and decreasing after expiration.

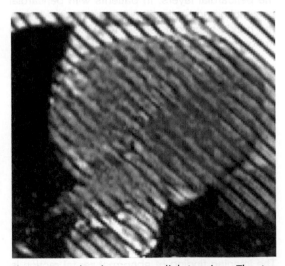

Fig. 8. Four-chamber myocardial tagging. The tag lines are bent but intact along the anterior pericardium, indicating abnormal myocardial-pericardial tethering. The lines normally break with cardiac motion (not shown).

Cardiac catheterization

This imaging technique can document the hemodynamics of constrictive physiology and can

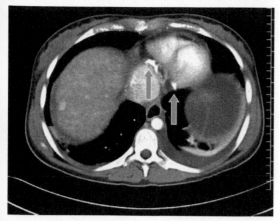

Fig. 9. Contrast-enhanced axial CT image. Note the coarse pericardial calcifications (*arrows*). This patient had undergone prior radiation therapy.

provide some discrimination between constrictive pericarditis and restrictive cardiomyopathy. Stroke volume is almost always reduced in constriction, primarily because of decreased diastolic filling. Pulmonary arterial and right ventricular systolic pressures are frequently increased in restrictive physiology, in the range of 35 to 45 mm Hg. This increase is not typical of constriction. Because of the physiologic changes caused by pericardial constriction, catheterization may reveal characteristic right atrial tracings, including a prominent Y descent and preserved X descent, in addition to an early and marked diastolic dip in biventricular pressures, the so-called dip-and-plateau or square-root sign.[10] The invasive nature of the procedure, as well as the exposure to ionizing radiation and potentially damaging iodinated contrast media, are among the potentially significant drawbacks to this imaging method.

Constrictive Pericarditis and Restrictive Cardiomyopathy

Restrictive cardiomyopathy is an uncommon cardiomyopathy characterized by abnormal stiffness of the ventricular myocardium.[10] Constrictive pericarditis and restrictive cardiomyopathy can have similar deleterious effects on the heart, most notably impaired ventricular filling in mid and late diastole with typically normal or near-normal systolic function, especially early in the disease process. In addition, although they may also appear similar clinically, the treatment of each involves different algorithms and tactics. Surgical pericardiectomy is the definitive treatment of constriction, whereas treatment of restrictive physiology is frequently targeted toward the underlying disease process, such as amyloidosis, which is the most common identifiable cause.[10] As stated earlier,

pericardial constriction often has classic MR imaging findings, including septal bounce and pericardial thickening/calcification. These findings are characteristically absent in restrictive cardiomyopathy, which usually shows thick-walled and rigid ventricles without the additional findings mentioned earlier. However, MR imaging is excellent at detecting all of these findings in both a noninvasive and nonirradiating way. Distinguishing between the two should guide clinicians toward the appropriate management strategy and, as a result, provide better outcomes for their patients.

SUMMARY

Pericardial constriction has many causes and is often a source of significant morbidity and mortality. Accurate diagnosis and differentiation from restrictive cardiomyopathy are vital to provide prompt and appropriate treatment. Pericardial imaging, particularly MR imaging, provides clinicians with comprehensive information about the pericardium and its effect on cardiac function, in addition to ancillary findings that may be missed by other modalities. However, multiple imaging techniques are often used in concert with clinical findings to provide a confident diagnosis.

REFERENCES

1. Yared K, Baggish AL, Picard MH, et al. Multimodality imaging of pericardial diseases. JACC Cardiovasc Imaging 2010;3(6):650–67.
2. Bogart J, Francone M. Pericardial disease: value of CT and MR imaging. Radiology 2013;267(2):340–56.
3. Leng H, Oh JK, Schaff HV, et al. Constrictive pericarditis in the modern era. Circulation 1999;100:1380–6.
4. Little W, Freeman G. Pericardial disease. Circulation 2006;113:1622–32.
5. Oh K, Shimizu M, Edwards WD, et al. Surgical pathology of the parietal pericardium. Cardiovasc Pathol 2001;10:157–68.
6. Deepak R, Edwards WD, Danielson GK, et al. Constrictive pericarditis in 26 patients with histologically normal parietal pericardium. Circulation 2003;108:1852–7.
7. Bogart J, Francone M. Cardiovascular magnetic resonance in pericardial disease. J Cardiovasc Magn Reson 2009;11:14.
8. Walker CM, Chung JH, Reddy GP. Septal Bounce. J Thorac Imaging 2012;27(1):1. JTI web-exclusive content.
9. Rajiah P. Cardiac MRI: part 2, pericardial diseases. AJR Am J Roentgenol 2011;197(4):W621–34.
10. Bonow RO, Mann DL, Zipes DP, et al. Braunwald's heart disease: a textbook of cardiovascular medicine. 9th edition. Elsevier; 2012.

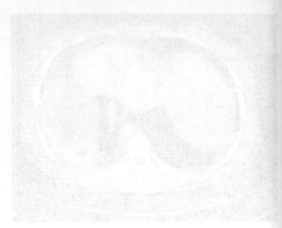

Prognostic Role of MR Imaging in Nonischemic Myocardial Disease

Kimberly Kallianos, MD[a], Gustavo L. Moraes, MD[b],
Karen G. Ordovas, MD, MAS[a],*

KEYWORDS

- Cardiac magnetic resonance • Delayed enhancement • Prognosis • Cardiomyopathy • Myocarditis
- Sarcoidosis • Amyloidosis

KEY POINTS

- An increasing body of data demonstrates that cardiac magnetic resonance (MR) imaging can provide prognostic information in a variety of nonischemic and diffuse myocardial diseases, including myocarditis, dilated and hypertrophic cardiomyopathies, sarcoidosis, amyloidosis, and arrhythmogenic right ventricular cardiomyopathy.
- Cardiac MR imaging can also supply incremental information above established clinical prognostic indicators, providing an additional tool for use in the prediction of disease progression, response to treatment, and risk stratification.

INTRODUCTION

The role of cardiac magnetic resonance (MR) imaging as a prognostic tool in patients with ischemic heart disease is well established, and MR imaging has been widely trusted in making clinical decisions regarding suitability for coronary revascularization. Recent efforts from the scientific imaging community have focused on the potential prognostic role of MR imaging biomarkers in patients with nonischemic myocardial diseases. In particular, delayed-enhancement cardiac MR imaging has been interrogated as a tool for risk stratification and treatment guidance in patients diagnosed with nonischemic cardiomyopathies and myocarditis. This article discusses current evidence on the role of MR imaging as a prognostic tool in these patients, with special focus on incremental value of cardiac MR imaging over well-established prognostic indicators.

MR IMAGING AS A PROGNOSTIC TOOL

The clinical research community has recently focused on trials to establish the use of MR imaging beyond a precise diagnostic tool, focusing on guidance of treatment strategies and identification of high-risk patients. Cardiac MR imaging can generate imaging biomarkers that have the potential to predict disease progression and patient response to specific treatment strategies, and to identify patients at risk for disease-specific mortality who may require more aggressive management. More importantly, MR imaging techniques for quantification of regional myocardial function and tissue characterization are able to identify

The authors have nothing to disclose.
[a] Department of Radiology and Biomedical Imaging, University of California, San Francisco, 350 Parnassus Avenue, San Francisco, CA 94117, USA; [b] Department of Radiology, Hospital Mae de Deus, R. José de Alencar, 286, Porto Alegre, Rio Grande do Sul 90110-270, Brazil
* Corresponding author.
E-mail address: Karen.Ordovas@ucsf.edu

Magn Reson Imaging Clin N Am 23 (2015) 89–94
http://dx.doi.org/10.1016/j.mric.2014.09.004

cardiac abnormalities at a subclinical stage, allowing for early interventions to prevent the development of symptomatic disease.

DISEASE-SPECIFIC CONSIDERATIONS
Myocarditis

In patients with viral myocarditis, the classic mortality predictors in clinical practice are related to severity of clinical symptoms, decreased systolic function, and left ventricular enlargement. These parameters are quantified using the New York Heart Association (NYHA) class, left ventricular ejection fraction (LVEF), and left ventricular end-diastolic volume index (LVEDVi), respectively.[1] In addition to providing accurate and reproducible quantification of LVEF and LVEDVi, MR imaging can demonstrate areas of abnormal signal on delayed-enhancement images, which have been associated with worse outcome in patients with myocarditis (**Fig. 1**). A recent study including 222 patients with biopsy-proven myocarditis and a follow-up of 4.7 years has shown that the presence of delayed enhancement has a hazard ratio of 12.8 for all-cause mortality and 8.4 for cardiac mortality.[2] In addition, this study showed that delayed-enhancement MR imaging had a hazard ratio significantly higher than that for LVEF, LVEDVi, and NYHA class. The presence of delayed enhancement has been described as a common feature in patients with chronic heart failure from myocarditis, supporting the hypothesis that the presence of scar on MR imaging is associated with worse clinical disease.[3]

Dilated Cardiomyopathy

Quantification of left ventricular systolic function, measured by LVEF, is a well-established indicator of prognosis in patients with nonischemic dilated cardiomyopathy, and can be precisely determined with volumetric cardiac MR imaging analysis.[4] It has been recently demonstrated that the presence of delayed enhancement on cardiac MR imaging also indicates a worse prognosis in patients with dilated cardiomyopathy (**Fig. 2**). Gulati and colleagues[5] have shown that patients with myocardial fibrosis on delayed-enhancement imaging have significantly higher mortality rate in comparison with patients without abnormalities on delayed-enhancement imaging, with a hazard ratio of 2.96 (95% confidence interval [CI] 1.87–4.69) and an absolute risk difference of 16.2% (95% CI 8.2%–24.2%). In addition, abnormal delayed-enhancement imaging had an incremental role in prognostication of patients with dilated cardiomyopathy when compared with LVEF alone, with a significant improvement in risk reclassification for all-cause mortality and a sudden cardiac death composite. Assomull and colleagues[6] have previously shown that the presence of mid-wall fibrosis in patients with dilated cardiomyopathy was associated with a higher rate of a predefined primary combined end point of all-cause mortality and hospitalization for a cardiovascular event (hazard ratio 3.4, $P = .01$), independently of ventricular remodeling.

In addition to delayed-enhancement imaging, dyssynchronous left ventricular contraction has also been interrogated as a prognostic tool in patients with dilated cardiomyopathy. Taylor and colleagues[7] have shown that combined MR imaging assessment of delayed enhancement and left ventricular dyssynchrony predicted response to cardiac resynchronization therapy (CRT) in 40 patients with cardiomyopathy and advanced heart failure. The investigators concluded that the concomitant assessment of scar and dyssynchrony is unique to MR imaging, and seems to be a reliable tool in predicting the response to CRT.

Hypertrophic Cardiomyopathy

Left ventricular mass has been recognized as the most important marker of disease severity and prognosis in patients with hypertrophic cardiomyopathy (HCM).[8] In current practice, patients with HCM are risk stratified based on the following combination of clinical and imaging criteria: family

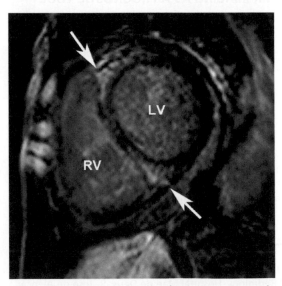

Fig. 1. Myocarditis. Delayed-enhancement image in the short-axis plane in a patient with viral myocarditis. Note the abnormal signal in the anteroseptal and inferoseptal left ventricular walls (*arrows*). LV, left ventricle; RV, right ventricle.

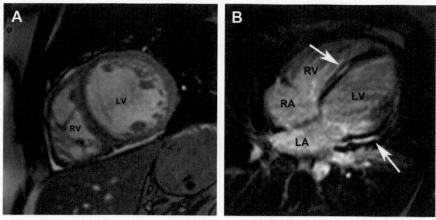

Fig. 2. Dilated cardiomyopathy. Steady-state free precession cine image in the short-axis plane (*A*) shows an enlarged left ventricle (LV) in a patient with dilated cardiomyopathy. Delayed-enhancement image in the horizontal long-axis plane (*B*) shows mid-wall enhancement in the septum and lateral wall (*arrows*), which has been associated with poor prognosis in these patients. LA, left atrium; RA, right atrium; RV, right ventricle.

history of major cardiac death; unexplained syncope; abnormal blood pressure response to exercise; nonsustained ventricular tachycardia; and severe left ventricular hypertrophy, defined as left ventricular wall thickness greater than or equal to 30 mm.[9] The 2003 American College of Cardiology (ACC)/European Society of Cardiology guidelines and the 2011 ACC Foundation/American Heart Association guidelines for diagnosis and treatment of hypertrophic cardiomyopathy recommend preventive implantable cardioverter-defibrillator (ICD) implantation in patients with at least 2 of these criteria, and the adoption of these guidelines in clinical practice has resulted in significant mortality reduction.[10] However, there is still suboptimal risk stratification for patients with intermediate risk based on current guidelines, for whom it is unclear if prophylactic pacemaker implantation is beneficial.

Recent imaging studies have indicated that the presence and extent of delayed gadolinium enhancement on cardiac MR imaging (**Fig. 3**) are strong predictors of inducible ventricular tachycardia and mortality in patients with HCM, independent of established prognostic markers. It has been shown that patients with hypertrophic cardiomyopathy and any degree of delayed enhancement have a 7-fold higher risk of nonsustained ventricular tachycardia on Holter monitoring in comparison with patients without the imaging

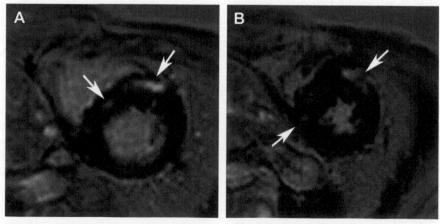

Fig. 3. Hypertrophic cardiomyopathy. Delayed-enhancement images in the short-axis plane at the base (*A*) and mid-ventricular (*B*) levels in a patient with hypertrophic cardiomyopathy presenting with arrhythmias. Abnormal enhancement is seen in the ventricular septum and in the anterior interventricular junction (*arrows*), with a mid-wall distribution. Note the asymmetric hypertrophy of the septum.

abnormality.[11] Bruder and colleagues[12] have also demonstrated that the presence of scar detected by delayed-enhancement MR imaging is an independent predictor of all-cause mortality and cardiac mortality in HCM patients (odds ratios of 5.47 for all-cause and 8.01 for cardiac mortality). A recent meta-analysis including more than 1000 patients with HCM, 60% of them with abnormal delayed enhancement on MR imaging, also reported that delayed enhancement is a significant predictor of all-cause mortality and cardiac mortality, with a pooled odds ratio of 4.4 and 2.9, respectively.[13] In addition, it has been shown that the extent of the delayed enhancement in patients with HCM is associated with progressive clinical disease.[14,15]

A potential important application of delayed-enhancement MR imaging is guiding management in patients with moderate left ventricular hypertrophy, mild blood pressure response to exercise, or some episodes of ventricular tachycardia, but who do not meet criteria for preventive ICD implantation based on current guidelines. However, prospective studies demonstrating the usefulness of MR imaging for guiding management in this particular population have not yet been interrogated in large clinical trials.

Sarcoidosis

There are limited data on the role of MR imaging for prognostic characterization in patients with cardiac sarcoidosis. The largest publication on this topic is a retrospective study including 61 patients with histologic diagnosis of cardiac sarcoidosis, who were followed clinically for approximately 100 months.[16] The investigators described an association between the presence of delayed enhancement and development of a composite outcome including ventricular arrhythmia, admission for heart failure, and mortality.

Amyloidosis

Delayed-enhancement imaging in patients with cardiac amyloidosis is very challenging given the lack of preserved areas of myocardium, which ultimately allow for characterization of areas with abnormal enhancement. The inversion-recovery sequence used for delayed-enhancement imaging relies on the differences in T1 relaxation between normal and abnormal myocardium. Nevertheless, Selvanayagam and colleagues[17] have described that the presence of global subendocardial myocardial delayed enhancement in patients with cardiac amyloidosis was associated with more extensive histologic amyloid deposition. Moreover, they demonstrated an association between the degree of delayed enhancement and markers of disease severity, including NYHA functional class, cardiac mass, ejection fraction, and electrocardiographic parameters.

To date there are limited data on the role of MR imaging as a predictor of mortality in patients with cardiac amyloidosis. Migrino and colleagues[18] studied 29 patients with cardiac amyloidosis for approximately 40 months and did not find an association between the presence of delayed enhancement and mortality. However, the cohort had only 5 adverse outcomes during the follow-up period.

It is plausible that, given the diffuse myocardial involvement in cardiac amyloidosis, areas of enhancement in delayed-enhancement imaging are likely not representative of the severity of disease, and therefore not a good marker of prognosis. MR imaging techniques capable of global tissue characterization, such as T1 and T2 mapping, may provide more reliable predictors of mortality in these patients.

Arrhythmogenic Right Ventricular Cardiomyopathy

Although the presence of delayed enhancement on cardiac MR imaging is not part of the diagnostic criteria for the diagnosis of arrhythmogenic right ventricular cardiomyopathy,[19] it has been described that the presence of right ventricular delayed enhancement is predictive of inducible ventricular tachycardia at programmed electric stimulation, suggesting a possible role of MR imaging in the prognostic assessment of these patients.[20]

PERSPECTIVES FOR CLINICAL PRACTICE

Understanding the value of MR imaging findings for prognostic characterization of patients with nonischemic cardiomyopathy is essential for imagers focused on providing patients the most benefit from an imaging test. In addition to providing standard cardiac reports, it is our role as imagers to highlight for clinicians disease-specific markers of poor prognosis. This advice includes, whenever relevant, quantitative information of ventricular volumes, global and regional ventricular function, myocardial mass, and extent of delayed enhancement. Generating clinically relevant reports will optimize the use of cardiac MR imaging as a diagnostic and prognostic tool, and has the potential to improve patients' outcomes.

SUMMARY

The role of cardiac MR imaging as a prognostic tool in patients with ischemic heart disease is well established. However, an increasing body of data now demonstrates that cardiac MR imaging can provide prognostic information through both evaluation of cardiac structural features and myocardial composition in a variety of nonischemic and diffuse myocardial diseases.

In myocarditis, the presence of myocardial delayed enhancement has a hazard ratio for both all-cause and cardiac mortality that is significantly higher than measures of left ventricular volume and NYHA classification. In both dilated and hypertrophic cardiomyopathy, the presence of delayed enhancement is associated with increased mortality risk. Specifically, in patients with dilated cardiomyopathy, abnormal delayed enhancement has an incremental prognostic role in comparison with LVEF, allowing improved risk stratification. In addition, cardiac MR imaging has a role in evaluating for CRT. Myocardial delayed enhancement has been shown to be an independent predictor of ventricular tachycardia and cardiac mortality in addition to all-cause mortality in patients with hypertrophic cardiomyopathy. Fewer data are available regarding the prognostic information provided by delayed myocardial enhancement in sarcoidosis and arrhythmogenic right ventricular dysplasia. Although there is no strong evidence that MR imaging is an important prognostic tool in patients with cardiac amyloidosis, advanced MR imaging techniques capable of global tissue characterization, such as T1 and T2 mapping, may allow mortality prediction in these patients.

In multiple cases, cardiac MR imaging provides incremental information in patients with diffuse and nonischemic myocardial disease, acting as an additional tool for use in prediction of disease progression, response to treatment, and risk stratification. In contrast to many clinical parameters, cardiac MR imaging allows quantification of regional and subclinical myocardial dysfunction, which may permit early intervention. Given these features, cardiac MR imaging has the potential to improve outcomes in patients with nonischemic myocardial diseases, and can be a valuable tool for prognostic characterization.

REFERENCES

1. Kindermann I, Kindermann M, Kandolf R, et al. Predictors of outcome in patients with suspected myocarditis. Circulation 2008;118:639–48.
2. Grun S, Schumm J, Greulich S, et al. Long-term follow-up of biopsy-proven viral myocarditis: predictors of mortality and incomplete recovery. J Am Coll Cardiol 2012;59(18):1604–15.
3. De Cobelli F, Pieroni M, Esposito A, et al. Delayed gadolinium-enhanced cardiac magnetic resonance in patients with chronic myocarditis presenting with heart failure or recurrent arrhythmias. J Am Coll Cardiol 2006;47(8):1649–54.
4. Curtis JP, Sokol SI, Wang Y, et al. The association of left ventricular ejection fraction, mortality, and cause of death in stable outpatients with heart failure. J Am Coll Cardiol 2003;42(4):736–42.
5. Gulati A, Jabbour A, Ismail TF, et al. Association of fibrosis with mortality and sudden cardiac death in patients with nonischemic dilated cardiomyopathy. JAMA 2013;309(9):896–908.
6. Assomull RG, Prasad SK, Lyne J, et al. Cardiovascular magnetic resonance, fibrosis, and prognosis in dilated cardiomyopathy. J Am Coll Cardiol 2006; 48(10):1977–85.
7. Taylor AJ, Elsik M, Broughton A, et al. Combined dyssynchrony and scar imaging with cardiac magnetic resonance imaging predicts clinical response and long-term prognosis following cardiac resynchronization therapy. Europace 2010;12(5):708–13.
8. Olivotto I, Maron MS, Autore C, et al. Assessment and significance of left ventricular mass by cardiovascular magnetic resonance in hypertrophic cardiomyopathy. J Am Coll Cardiol 2008;52(7): 559–66.
9. Gersh BJ, Maron BJ, Bonow RO, et al. 2011 ACCF/ AHA guideline for the diagnosis and treatment of hypertrophic cardiomyopathy: executive summary: a report of the American College of Cardiology Foundation/American Heart Association Task Force on Practice Guidelines. J Am Coll Cardiol 2011; 58(25):2703–38.
10. O'Mahony C, Tome-Esteban M, Lambiase PD, et al. A validation study of the 2003 American College of Cardiology/European Society of Cardiology and 2011 American College of Cardiology Foundation/ American Heart Association risk stratification and treatment algorithms for sudden cardiac death in patients with hypertrophic cardiomyopathy. Heart 2013;99(8):534–41.
11. Adabag AS, Maron BJ, Applebaum E, et al. Occurrence and frequency of arrhythmias in hypertrophic cardiomyopathy in relation to delayed enhancement on cardiovascular magnetic resonance. J Am Coll Cardiol 2008;51(14):1369–74.
12. Bruder O, Wagner A, Jensen CJ, et al. Myocardial scar visualized by cardiovascular magnetic resonance imaging predicts major adverse events in patients with hypertrophic cardiomyopathy. J Am Coll Cardiol 2010;56(11):875–87.
13. Green JJ, Berger JS, Kramer CM, et al. Prognostic value of late gadolinium enhancement in clinical outcomes for hypertrophic cardiomyopathy. JACC Cardiovasc Imaging 2012;5(4):370–7.
14. Moon JC, Reed E, Sheppard MN, et al. The histologic basis of late gadolinium enhancement cardiovascular magnetic resonance in hypertrophic

cardiomyopathy. J Am Coll Cardiol 2004;43(12): 2260–4.

15. Moon JC, McKenna WJ, McCrohon JA, et al. Toward clinical risk assessment in hypertrophic cardiomyopathy with gadolinium cardiovascular magnetic resonance. J Am Coll Cardiol 2003; 41(9):1561–7.

16. Shafee MA, Fukuda K, Wakayama Y, et al. Delayed enhancement on cardiac magnetic resonance imaging is a poor prognostic factor in patients with cardiac sarcoidosis. J Cardiol 2012;60(6):448–53.

17. Selvanayagam JB, Leong DP. MR imaging and cardiac amyloidosis: where to go from here? JACC Cardiovasc Imaging 2010;3(2):165–7.

18. Migrino RQ, Christenson R, Szabo A, et al. Prognostic implication of late gadolinium enhancement in cardiac MRI on light chain (AL) amyloidosis on long term follow up. BMC Med Phys 2009;9:5.

19. Marcus FI, McKenna WJ, Sherrill D, et al. Diagnosis of arrhythmogenic right ventricular cardiomyopathy/dysplasia: proposed modification of the Task Force Criteria. Eur Heart J 2010;31(7):806–14.

20. Tandri H, Saranathan M, Rodriguez RE, et al. Noninvasive detection of myocardial fibrosis in arrhythmogenic right ventricular cardiomyopathy using delayed-enhancement magnetic resonance imaging. J Am Coll Cardiol 2005;45(1):98–103.

PET/MR Imaging
Current and Future Applications for Cardiovascular Disease

David M. Naeger, MD*, Spencer C. Behr, MD

KEYWORDS

- Cardiac PET/MR hybrid imaging • [¹⁸F] Fluorodeoxyglucose • Myocardial perfusion stress tests

KEY POINTS

- Combined PET/magnetic resonance (MR) systems are being developed and refined, with many commercially available systems now entering the market.
- Cardiac indications are potentially a fruitful area for this new technology, given how important PET and MR imaging each are in the workup and management of various cardiac diseases.
- Research to define the most effective use of this new hybrid technology is at a very early stage, although many preliminary studies have been promising.

INTRODUCTION

Several different imaging modalities have been used to study the heart, each with strengths and weaknesses. Two advanced imaging modalities, magnetic resonance (MR) imaging and PET, have enjoyed decades of clinical use, each evolving to become integral to the management of certain cardiac patients.

MR imaging offers the ability to evaluate cardiac anatomy with high resolution and detailed tissue characterization. High temporal resolution cine image sequences have been developed, which capture high-resolution images of the heart throughout the cardiac cycle. Blood flow can be visualized and measured via velocity-encoded cine sequences. Postcontrast imaging adds an additional dimension, allowing for angiographic evaluation and assessment of early and late myocardial enhancement. Advanced MR techniques continue to be developed, including MR spectroscopy and sequences capable of measuring myocardial strain, T1 mapping, and so forth. The full range of cardiac MR sequences, all providing targeted information, is available without the use of ionizing radiation.

Independently, PET has also become a modality ubiquitously used in cardiac imaging. Myocardial perfusion, historically evaluated via single-photon emission computed tomography (SPECT) tracers, can be assessed using PET agents. Rubidium-82 (Rb-82) and nitrogen-13 (N-13) ammonia allow for high-resolution imaging in a short acquisition time, and the possibility of quantitative measurements of coronary artery blood flow. These agents require an on-site generator or cyclotron, respectively, owing to the short half-life of these agents. Fluorine-18 [¹⁸F]-based perfusion agents, which have a longer half-life and can be transported

The authors have nothing to disclose.
Department of Radiology and Biomedical Imaging, University of California, San Francisco, 505 Parnassus Avenue, M-391, Box 0628, San Francisco, CA 94143-0628, USA
* Corresponding author.
E-mail address: david.naeger@ucsf.edu

Magn Reson Imaging Clin N Am 23 (2015) 95–103
http://dx.doi.org/10.1016/j.mric.2014.09.006
1064-9689/15/$ – see front matter © 2015 Elsevier Inc. All rights reserved.

over greater distances, are in late-stage clinical trials. An approved ^{18}F perfusion agent could potentially result in PET replacing SPECT as the first-line modality for imaging myocardial perfusion. [18]F tagged to glucose ([^{18}F]–fluorodeoxyglucose [FDG]) has been used to evaluate the myocardium in several settings, including conditions involving inflammation of the myocardium.

PET/computed tomography (CT) and SPECT/CT hybrid technologies have demonstrated the power of hybrid nuclear medicine imaging, with PET/CT in particular revolutionizing oncologic imaging. MR has several advantages over CT, making it potentially an excellent complement to the molecular information provided by PET, including excellent soft-tissue contrast, advanced functional techniques, and lack of ionization radiation. Combined PET/MR hybrid systems, however, have been an elusive technological goal until recently. MR imaging requires a bulky electromagnet and a plethora of electronics while PET cameras require a large array of sensitive detectors. The immense technological limitations of merging these technologies have finally been overcome in commercially viable scanners.

The clinical value of PET/MR as a hybrid technology has only limitedly been evaluated thus far. The published literature regarding this technology for cardiac indications, in particular, is somewhat limited. Cardiac indications would prima facie seem like a fruitful area, given the unique and complementary strengths of each modality individually.[1,2] In its simplest form, PET/MR could offer "one-stop shop" imaging modality for patients in whom PET and MR studies are separately indicated. For indications whereby acquiring both sets of images could theoretically be complementary, though not currently the standard of care, the new-found ease of acquiring both sets of images via hybrid scanners may result in a hybrid evaluation becoming the new standard. Finally, future research may determine ways to more deeply integrate the information obtained from each modality, resulting in new levels of diagnostic information.

This article reviews of the current state of PET/MR technology, followed by a brief overview of cardiac indications for which PET/MR may hold great promise.

INSTRUMENTATION

Several technical challenges had to be overcome in designing commercially viable PET/MR imaging systems. A variety of solutions have been developed. The most straightforward solution, a sequential system, involves the installation of a PET/CT scanner and an MR scanner adjacent to each other, in line, connected by a single patient table.[3] Sequential systems can also be installed with the 2 scanners in separate rooms, joined by a table system that spans the 2 rooms.[4] Both of these designs require relatively minimal changes to the underlying scanners, although they require large installation footprints. In addition, a truly simultaneous acquisition of PET and MR data is not possible.

The most integrated of the PET/MR designs is a concurrent system, in which the PET and MR components are physically combined in one scanner with a single gantry (**Fig. 1**).[5] This design involves a significant redesign of both the MR and PET hardware, most notably redesigning the MR hardware to make room for the PET and altering the PET detectors to become less sensitive to the MR scanner's magnetic fields. Fully integrated systems have smaller footprints, and allow for the simultaneous acquisition of PET and MR data. Simultaneous image acquisition allows for the most flexibility in designing optimal imaging studies.

PET/MR systems must have a mechanism to address attenuation correction, another major obstacle faced when developing these systems for clinical use. PET-only scanners and PET/CT systems use built-in radionuclide sources and CT, respectively, to create attenuation maps; neither technology is available in PET/MR

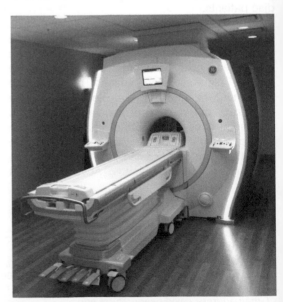

Fig. 1. A fully integrated PET/magnetic resonance system by General Electric Healthcare.

systems. Several methods to address attenuation correction have been studied including template-based methods,[6–8] atlas-based methods,[6,9,10] and approaches based on MR image segmentation,[6,7,11–13] and PET emission.[14–16] Future studies will likely determine which approach is the most optimal.

Hybrid PET studies are limited by patient motion. First, patient motion can result in misregistration between the anatomic and PET images. With potentially longer acquisition times, PET/MR may suffer from more misregistration issues in comparison with PET/CT. Second, patient motion can degrade the PET images themselves, given that PET images are acquired over multiple minutes per imaging bed. This limitation is particularly problematic when imaging the heart because of cardiac and respiratory motion, which can result in 4.9 to 9 mm of movement.[17,18] PET/MR systems, however, unlike PET/CT systems, have the potential to correct PET data for patient motion. Cine MR imaging can demonstrate the full range of cardiac and respiratory motion, thereby allowing for a map to be created that can be applied to the raw PET data to correct for motion.[19]

CARDIAC TUMORS

The evaluation of cardiac tumors may be the most straightforward potential application of combined PET/MR scanners. CT is fairly limited in the evaluation of cardiac tumors, whereas MR imaging provides far more detail with regard to tissue characterization and the evaluation of tissue planes.

In the case of malignant cardiac tumors, PET is often indicated for staging purposes, owing to the improved sensitivity of PET for metastatic disease in comparison with anatomic imaging alone. PET is also often used for the evaluation of treatment effectiveness and for surveillance.

When both anatomic and metabolic imaging is indicated in the evaluation of a cardiac tumor, PET/MR may be superior to PET/CT. The primary tumor almost certainly would be more clearly demonstrated by MR imaging, and even in the evaluation for nodal and metastatic disease, PET/MR would likely be similar or superior to PET/CT.[20] Although this supposition has not specifically assessed for cardiac malignancies, several studies have reported on the value of PET/MR in comparison with PET/CT for a variety of other tumors, including lung cancer.[21] One notable weakness of PET/MR is in the evaluation of the lungs.

MYOCARDIAL ISCHEMIA AND INFARCTION

The extent of patients' coronary artery disease (CAD) can be evaluated by cardiac MR imaging, although the modality is not considered first line for this indication. First-pass perfusion with gadolinium can demonstrate perfusion defects at stress and rest, analogous to nuclear perfusion studies.[22] Direct coronary artery imaging is also possible by MR imaging,[23] although coronary CT angiography is currently the noninvasive gold standard owing to its high resolution and fast acquisition times.

Cardiac MR imaging is more commonly used in the evaluation of myocardial infarctions. Late gadolinium enhancement (LGE) is demonstrated in acute and chronic infarctions, with the contrast being retained in the expanded extracellular in necrotic myocardium early and in regions of fibrosis later.

Myocardial perfusion with PET tracers such as N-13 ammonia and Rb-82 is used more commonly than MR imaging to evaluate for CAD (**Fig. 2**). PET perfusion studies have high sensitivity and specificity for the evaluation of obstructive CAD,[24–26] and the PET data can also be processed to quantify coronary artery blood flow. This assessment is of particular value in patients with balanced ischemia, which can be underappreciated on visual evaluation.[27,28]

Like cardiac MR imaging, infarctions may also be demonstrated by PET. Myocardial infarctions on PET imaging are seen as matched perfusion defects on both rest and stress, although hibernating myocardium can have a similar appearance.

Hybrid PET/MR systems may be particularly well suited for the evaluation of patients with suspected CAD and/or infarctions. Specifically, the strengths of MR imaging and PET each could theoretically complement weaknesses in the other, all with the ease of a single imaging session.[29] In particular, fully integrated systems may allow for simultaneous PET and MR acquisition after a single administration of a myocardial stress agent. Most intriguingly, perhaps, is the ability to evaluate for CAD/infarctions (relying heavily on the PET images) and viable myocardium (relying mostly on the MR images) in one session. Assessing for viability by PET usually requires the administration of a different radiotracer (FDG) than those used for perfusion; MR imaging only requires the administration of gadolinium (see later discussion).

Another potential application for combined PET/MR systems is the differentiation of ischemic and nonischemic cardiomyopathies. At present, PET

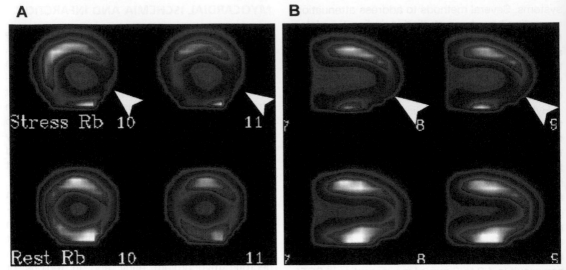

Fig. 2. Reduced myocardial perfusion during stress: Short-axis (*A*) and vertical long-axis (*B*) images from an Rb-82 stress (*top rows*) and rest (*bottom rows*) myocardial perfusion PET study show an inferolateral wall (*white arrowheads*) reversible perfusion defect in a 79-year-old man who presented for preoperative clearance before lumbar laminectomy.

and MR both provide imperfect information to differentiate between the two. PET can identify areas of decreased perfusion, areas of viability, and regions at risk, while MR is excellent at assessing myocardial scarring and functional information. The simultaneous acquisition of PET and MR data may allow for a more accurate overall assessment.

VIABILITY

Cardiac MR imaging suggests viable myocardium when nonenhancing myocardium is seen adjacent to subendocardial infarcts on late gadolinium enhancement sequences. No special patient preparation is needed, and the sequences used are the same that identify the necrotic myocardium and scar.

PET suggests viable myocardium when FDG uptake is demonstrated in regions of fixed, decreased perfusion (**Fig. 3**). PET is widely considered the gold standard for assessing for viable myocardium that could benefit from revascularization.[30–32] In repetitively stunned or chronic hypoperfused myocardium, anaerobic metabolism is favored, which results in the elevated glucose uptake visualized with FDG. Conversely, scarred myocardium shows absent perfusion and absent FDG uptake (**Fig. 4**).

Simultaneous PET/MR acquisition has the potential of merging these two powerful techniques into one. The molecular information of FDG PET combined with the structural and functional

information obtained from MR may add additional diagnostic sensitivity or specificity. In hybrid PET/MR studies in which only perfusion agents are administered for the PET, the MR evaluation could preferentially provide information about possible viability.

SARCOIDOSIS

Cardiac sarcoidosis, a potentially fatal disease in which noncaseating, nonnecrotic granulomas develop in the myocardium, may be particularly well suited for imaging with hybrid PET/MR systems.[33]

Cardiac MR imaging can reveal the active inflammation phase of sarcoidosis. Focal wall thickening, focal wall motion abnormalities, increased signal intensity on T2-weighted images, and early gadolinium enhancement[34] can all be seen in this phase. Fibrosis, seen in the chronic phase of the disease, is demonstrated by late gadolinium enhancement.[35] Overlap of these 2 phases and, therefore, overlap of these imaging patterns, is possible.

PET also demonstrates abnormalities in the inflammation and fibrotic phases of sarcoidosis. FDG uptake suggests inflammation (**Fig. 5**),[36] which notably relies on glucose uptake, rather than the mechanisms indirectly imaged by MR imaging (edema, expanded extracellular space, and so forth). Myocardial fibrosis is demonstrated on PET perfusion studies, usually as focal perfusion defects.[37] The PET evaluation of sarcoidosis with

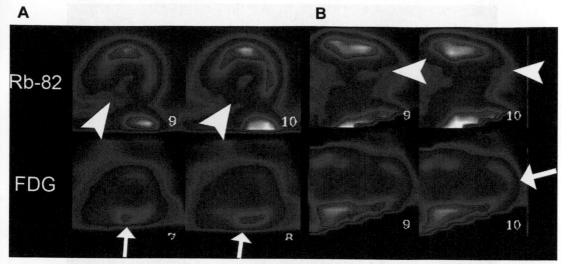

Fig. 3. Viable myocardium: Short-axis (*A*) and vertical long-axis (*B*) images from resting Rb-82 PET (*top rows*) and [^{18}F] fluorodeoxyglucose (FDG) PET viability study (*bottom rows*) in a 56-year-old man with a history of endocarditis and severe mitral valve regurgitation. The patient originally presented with severe cardiogenic shock and was found to have a large fixed perfusion defect at another hospital (not shown). Perfusion images show a large, severe defect involving the distal inferior wall and much of the apex (*white arrowheads*). These regions demonstrated moderate FDG uptake on the select short-axis images and subtle FDG uptake in the apex on the selected vertical long-axis images (*white arrows*), compatible with regions of viable myocardium.

FDG requires a patient preparation that suppresses normal use of myocardial glucose. A variety of preparations have been proposed with varying success, including prolonged fasting,[38] high-fat low-carbohydrate diets,[39] and the administration of intravenous nonfractionated heparin.[36,38] In addition, PET suffers from a somewhat lower spatial resolution than MR imaging.

Although a clear gold standard is lacking in making the diagnosis of cardiac sarcoidosis, PET and MR imaging both appear to have imperfect sensitivity and specificity, most notably with PET demonstrating a relatively weaker specificity.[40] Because PET and MR imaging rely on different underlying mechanisms in this disease, the combination of the two could increase the overall diagnostic accuracy.[33,41]

MYOCARDITIS

Other causes of myocardial inflammation also demonstrate abnormalities on PET and MR imaging. Myocarditis resulting from infection, autoimmune mechanisms, toxin exposure, allergic reactions, or idiopathic causes can result in hyperemia, edema, wall motion abnormalities, necrosis, and fibrosis. These pathophysiologic processes can be visualized by MR imaging. Indeed, diagnostic criteria using MR imaging findings have been published.[42] FDG PET has less

extensively been studied in the evaluation of myocarditis, although increased FDG uptake has been described in this setting. Ozawa and colleagues[43] described overall moderate sensitivity and good specificity in demonstrating the inflammation of myocarditis via FDG PET in a comparison with endomyocardial biopsy. Imaging within 2 weeks of symptom onset demonstrated particularly high sensitivity and specificity. Studies of simultaneous PET/MR imaging for this indication have not been published thus far, although this is a potential area of interest.

OTHER POTENTIAL APPLICATIONS AND FUTURE DIRECTIONS

PET and MR technology is likely to continue to advance, particularly with large improvements expected in combined systems. New contrast agents and radiotracers also hold the promise of new applications for stand-alone and combined PET/MR systems. Already a multitude of PET tracers are at various stages of development, including tracers that localize to regions of apoptosis, hypoxia, protein synthesis, DNA synthesis, and angiogenesis. Some investigators have even been developing dual-modality agents that contain both a radionuclide and magnetic nanoparticles.[44,45]

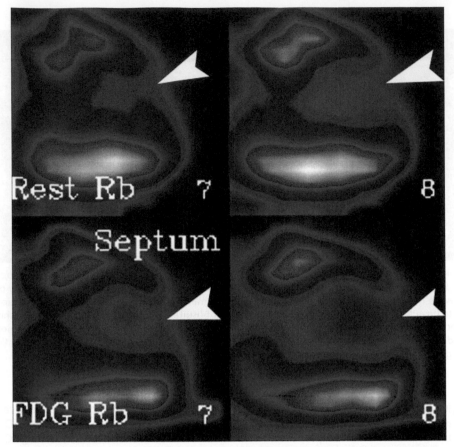

Fig. 4. Myocardial scarring from a myocardial infarction: Vertical long-axis images from an Rb-82 rest (*top row*) myocardial perfusion PET study show a large anterior wall perfusion defect that extends into the apex (*top white arrow heads*). The FDG viability PET study (*bottom row*) shows a matched metabolic defect (*bottom white arrow heads*), confirming scarring in this 54-year-old man with history of 3-vessel disease and multiple prior coronary artery stents who presented with decreased ejection fraction and a nonreversible perfusion defect on prior myocardial stress test (not shown).

Future research in the following areas may yield new uses for combined PET/MR systems:

- Atherosclerosis: With improved special resolution, MR could potentially evaluate the content of plaques while PET tracers could assess the degree of plaque inflammation,[46] factors that could indicate plaques at risk for rupture.
- Stem cell engraftment: PET/MR may be an optimal imaging system for demonstration of stem cell engraftment.[45,47]
- Sympathetic imaging: Radionuclides such as iodine-124 metaiodobenzylguanidine can be used to assess myocardial sympathetic innervation defects in a variety of conditions, including heart failure.[48]
- Remodeling after myocardial infarction: PET and MR together may optimally identify inflammation in infarcted myocardium, which may reflect increased risk of adverse remodeling.[49,50]

LIMITATIONS OF HYBRID PET/MAGNETIC RESONANCE IMAGING

Although there are many enticing features of PET/MR systems, several significant factors could hamper its widespread acceptance into routine clinical care, including:

- Situations in which CT remains superior, including presently the evaluation of the lungs and the coronary arteries.
- Imaging patients with implanted electronic devices or other contraindications to MR imaging. Such devices are common in cardiac patients.
- Imaging patients with severe renal impairment or renal failure, who generally cannot receive gadolinium.
- At present many issues surrounding scheduling, reporting, and billing have yet to be worked out for combined PET/MR studies, which can hinder adoption of this technology in the short term.

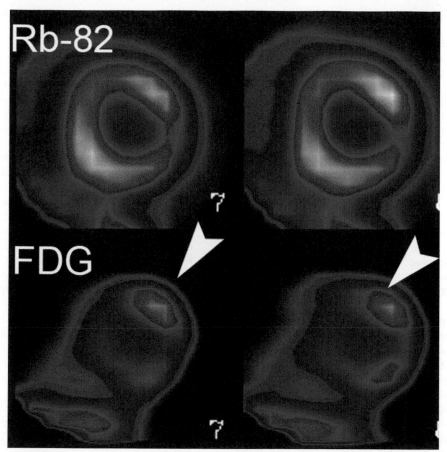

Fig. 5. Active myocardial sarcoidosis: Short-axis rest Rb-82 (*top row*) and FDG (*bottom row*) PET images from a 35-year-old woman with palpitations and syncope and suspected cardiac sarcoidosis. FDG PET images, which are presented at a slightly lower magnification, show patchy areas of FDG uptake most prominent in the antero-lateral wall (*white arrowheads*), suggesting a region of active sarcoidosis. No significant perfusion defect is apparent on this slice (nor on the remaining short-axis slices, not shown), which argues against any significant scarring resulting from chronic cardiac sarcoidosis.

REFERENCES

1. Nekolla SG, Martinez-Moeller A, Saraste A. PET and MRI in cardiac imaging: from validation studies to integrated applications. Eur J Nucl Med Mol Imaging 2009;36(Suppl 1):S121–30.
2. Rischpler C, Nekolla SG, Dregely I, et al. Hybrid PET/MR imaging of the heart: potential, initial experiences, and future prospects. J Nucl Med 2013; 54(3):402–15.
3. Zaidi H, Ojha N, Morich M, et al. Design and performance evaluation of a whole-body Ingenuity TF PET-MRI system. Phys Med Biol 2011;56(10):3091–106.
4. Veit-Haibach P, Kuhn FP, Wiesinger F, et al. PET-MR imaging using a tri-modality PET/CT-MR system with a dedicated shuttle in clinical routine. MAGMA 2013; 26(1):25–35.
5. Catana C, Guimaraes AR, Rosen BR. PET and MR imaging: the odd couple or a match made in heaven? J Nucl Med 2013;54(5):815–24.
6. Malone IB, Ansorge RE, Williams GB, et al. Attenuation correction methods suitable for brain imaging with a PET/MRI scanner: a comparison of tissue atlas and template attenuation map approaches. J Nucl Med 2011;52(7):1142–9.
7. Rota Kops E, Herzog H. Alternative methods for attenuation correction for PET images in MR-PET scanners. IEEE Nucl Sci Conf R 2007;6:4327–30.
8. Rota Kops E, Herzog H. Template-based attenuation correction for PET in MR-PET scanners. IEEE Nucl Sci Conf R 2008;3786–9.
9. Hofmann M, Steinke F, Scheel V, et al. MRI-based attenuation correction for PET/MRI: a novel approach combining pattern recognition and atlas registration. J Nucl Med 2008;49(11):1875–83.
10. Schreibmann E, Nye JA, Schuster DM, et al. MR-based attenuation correction for hybrid PET-MR brain imaging systems using deformable image registration. Med Phys 2010;37(5):2101–9.

11. Huang SC, Carson RE, Phelps ME, et al. A boundary method for attenuation correction in positron computed tomography. J Nucl Med 1981;22(7): 627–37.

12. Rota Kops E, Wagenkncht G, Scheins J, et al. Attenuation correction in MR-PET scanners with segmented T1-weighted MR images. IEEE Nucl Sci Conf R 2009;2530–3.

13. Wagenknecht G, Rota Kops E, Kaffanke J, et al. CT-based evaluation of segmented head regions for attenuation correction in MR-PET systems. IEEE Nucl Sci Conf R 2010;2793–7.

14. Martinez-Moller A, Souvatzoglou M, Navab N, et al. Artifacts from misaligned CT in cardiac perfusion PET/CT studies: frequency, effects, and potential solutions. J Nucl Med 2007;48(2):188–93.

15. Nuyts J, Bal G, Kehren F, et al. Completion of a truncated attenuation image from the attenuated PET emission data. IEEE Trans Med Imaging 2013; 32(2):237–46.

16. Nuyts J, Dupont P, Stroobants S, et al. Simultaneous maximum a posteriori reconstruction of attenuation and activity distributions from emission sinograms. IEEE Trans Med Imaging 1999;18(5):393–403.

17. Blume M, Martinez-Moller A, Keil A, et al. Joint reconstruction of image and motion in gated positron emission tomography. IEEE Trans Med Imaging 2010;29(11):1892–906.

18. Boucher L, Rodrigue S, Lecomte R, et al. Respiratory gating for 3-dimensional PET of the thorax: feasibility and initial results. J Nucl Med 2004; 45(2):214–9.

19. Ouyang J, Li Q, El Fakhri G. Magnetic resonance-based motion correction for positron emission tomography imaging. Semin Nucl Med 2013;43(1): 60–7.

20. Al-Nabhani KZ, Syed R, Michopoulou S, et al. Qualitative and quantitative comparison of PET/CT and PET/MR imaging in clinical practice. J Nucl Med 2014;55(1):88–94.

21. Yoon SH, Goo JM, Lee SM, et al. Positron emission tomography/magnetic resonance imaging evaluation of lung cancer: current status and future prospects. J Thorac Imaging 2014;29(1):4–16.

22. Kawel-Boehm N, Bremerich J. Magnetic resonance stress imaging of myocardial perfusion and wall motion. J Thorac Imaging 2014;29(1):30–7.

23. Kim WY, Danias PG, Stuber M, et al. Coronary magnetic resonance angiography for the detection of coronary stenoses. N Engl J Med 2001;345(26): 1863–9.

24. Klocke FJ, Baird MG, Lorell BH, et al. ACC/AHA/ASNC guidelines for the clinical use of cardiac radionuclide imaging—executive summary: a report of the American College of Cardiology/American Heart Association Task Force on practice guidelines (ACC/AHA/ASNC Committee to revise the 1995

guidelines for the clinical use of cardiac radionuclide imaging). J Am Coll Cardiol 2003;42(7): 1318–33.

25. McArdle BA, Dowsley TF, deKemp RA, et al. Does rubidium-82 PET have superior accuracy to SPECT perfusion imaging for the diagnosis of obstructive coronary disease?: a systematic review and meta-analysis. J Am Coll Cardiol 2012;60(18):1828–37.

26. Parker MW, Iskandar A, Limone B, et al. Diagnostic accuracy of cardiac positron emission tomography versus single photon emission computed tomography for coronary artery disease: a bivariate meta-analysis. Circ Cardiovasc Imaging 2012;5(6):700–7.

27. Kajander SA, Joutsiniemi E, Saraste M, et al. Clinical value of absolute quantification of myocardial perfusion with (15)O-water in coronary artery disease. Circ Cardiovasc Imaging 2011;4(6):678–84.

28. Parkash R, deKemp RA, Ruddy TD, et al. Potential utility of rubidium 82 PET quantification in patients with 3-vessel coronary artery disease. J Nucl Cardiol 2004;11(4):440–9.

29. Nensa F, Poeppel TD, Beiderwellen K, et al. Hybrid PET/MR imaging of the heart: feasibility and initial results. Radiology 2013;268(2):366–73.

30. Schinkel AF, Bax JJ, Poldermans D, et al. Hibernating myocardium: diagnosis and patient outcomes. Curr Probl Cardiol 2007;32(7):375–410.

31. Tillisch J, Brunken R, Marshall R, et al. Reversibility of cardiac wall-motion abnormalities predicted by positron tomography. N Engl J Med 1986;314(14): 884–8.

32. vom Dahl J, Eitzman DT, al-Aouar ZR, et al. Relation of regional function, perfusion, and metabolism in patients with advanced coronary artery disease undergoing surgical revascularization. Circulation 1994;90(5):2356–66.

33. Schneider S, Batrice A, Rischpler C, et al. Utility of multimodal cardiac imaging with PET/MRI in cardiac sarcoidosis: implications for diagnosis, monitoring and treatment. Eur Heart J 2013;35(5):312.

34. Schatka I, Bengel FM. Advanced imaging of cardiac sarcoidosis. J Nucl Med 2014;55(1):99–106.

35. Tadamura E, Yamamuro M, Kubo S, et al. Effectiveness of delayed enhanced MRI for identification of cardiac sarcoidosis: comparison with radionuclide imaging. AJR Am J Roentgenol 2005;185(1):110–5.

36. Ishimaru S, Tsujino I, Takei T, et al. Focal uptake on ^{18}F-fluoro-2-deoxyglucose positron emission tomography images indicates cardiac involvement of sarcoidosis. Eur Heart J 2005;26(15):1538–43.

37. Yamagishi H, Shirai N, Takagi M, et al. Identification of cardiac sarcoidosis with (13)N-NH(3)/(18)F-FDG PET. J Nucl Med 2003;44(7):1030–6.

38. Morooka M, Moroi M, Uno K, et al. Long fasting is effective in inhibiting physiological myocardial ^{18}F-FDG uptake and for evaluating active lesions of cardiac sarcoidosis. EJNMMI Res 2014;4:1–11.

39. Harisankar CN, Mittal BR, Agrawal KL, et al. Utility of high fat and low carbohydrate diet in suppressing myocardial FDG uptake. J Nucl Cardiol 2011;18(5):926–36.

40. Ohira H, Tsujino I, Ishimaru S, et al. Myocardial imaging with ^{18}F-fluoro-2-deoxyglucose positron emission tomography and magnetic resonance imaging in sarcoidosis. Eur J Nucl Med Mol Imaging 2008; 35(5):933–41.

41. Campbell P, Stewart GC, Padera RF, et al. Evaluation for cardiac sarcoidosis—uncertainty despite contemporary multi-modality imaging. J Card Fail 2010; 16(8):S107.

42. Friedrich MG, Marcotte F. Cardiac magnetic resonance assessment of myocarditis. Circ Cardiovasc Imaging 2013;6(5):833–9.

43. Ozawa K, Funabashi N, Daimon M, et al. Determination of optimum periods between onset of suspected acute myocarditis and (1)(8)F-fluorodeoxyglucose positron emission tomography in the diagnosis of inflammatory left ventricular myocardium. Int J Cardiol 2013;169(3):196–200.

44. Jarrett BR, Gustafsson B, Kukis DL, et al. Synthesis of ^{64}Cu-labeled magnetic nanoparticles for multimodal imaging. Bioconjug Chem 2008;19(7): 1496–504.

45. Higuchi T, Anton M, Dumler K, et al. Combined reporter gene PET and iron oxide MRI for monitoring survival and localization of transplanted cells in the rat heart. J Nucl Med 2009;50(7):1088–94.

46. Rudd JH, Warburton EA, Fryer TD, et al. Imaging atherosclerotic plaque inflammation with [18F]-fluorodeoxyglucose positron emission tomography. Circulation 2002;105(23):2708–11.

47. Zhang WY, Ebert AD, Narula J, et al. Imaging cardiac stem cell therapy: translations to human clinical studies. J Cardiovasc Transl Res 2011;4(4):514–22.

48. Bengel FM, Schwaiger M. Assessment of cardiac sympathetic neuronal function using PET imaging. J Nucl Cardiol 2004;11(5):603–16.

49. Lee WW, Marinelli B, van der Laan AM, et al. PET/MRI of inflammation in myocardial infarction. J Am Coll Cardiol 2012;59(2):153–63.

50. van der Laan AM, Nahrendorf M, Piek JJ. Healing and adverse remodelling after acute myocardial infarction: role of the cellular immune response. Heart 2012;98(18):1384–90.

Cardiovascular MR Imaging in Cardio-oncology

Ashenafi M. Tamene, MD[a], Carolina Masri, MD[b],
Suma H. Konety, MD, MS[a],*

KEYWORDS

- Cardio-oncology • Cardiotoxicity • Radiation-induced heart disease
- Cardiovascular magnetic resonance imaging

KEY POINTS

- Patients with cancer are at risk for developing short-term and long-term adverse cardiovascular outcomes, due to both direct and indirect off-target effects of cancer treatment.
- Cardiac magnetic resonance (CMR) imaging provides accurate assessment of left ventricular ejection fraction and should be used for monitoring cardiac function of patients both during and after cancer therapy.
- CMR imaging can additionally evaluate for myocardial, valvular, pericardial abnormalities; assess vascular compliance and provide tissue characterization of cardiac masses.

INTRODUCTION

Based on currently available estimates, there are 13.7 million patients with a history of cancer in the United States who are either cancer free or undergoing treatment, and about 1.7 million new cases are expected to be diagnosed in 2014.[1] Owing to significant progress made in diagnostic and treatment capabilities over the past few decades, a sizable proportion of these individuals have an increased chance of long-term survival.[1] Like diabetes or hypertension, cancer may now be considered as a chronic manageable disease and as such it requires not only early detection, periodic surveillance, and appropriate therapy but also control of comorbid conditions.[2] Cardio-oncology has emerged as a unique interface between the two fields, because cardiovascular events are increasingly being recognized as major sources of morbidity and mortality in cancer survivors, because of either direct cardiac toxicity of chemotherapeutic agents[2] or the presence of underlying concomitant cardiovascular comorbidities.[3,4]

Cancer can affect the cardiovascular system in multiple ways ranging from direct invasion of cardiac structures from primary or metastatic tumors of the heart to short-term or long-term cardiotoxic effects of treatment modalities, such as chemotherapy and radiation. The traditional focus of cardiac imaging has been on monitoring baseline and posttreatment left ventricular ejection fraction (LVEF), mostly through the use of echocardiography or multiple gated acquisition nuclear scans.[5] Cardiac magnetic resonance (CMR) imaging, by virtue of its accurate depiction of cardiac morphology and function, is rapidly being adopted as an imaging modality that can provide a comprehensive assessment in cardio-oncology (Fig. 1).[6]

Disclosure: The authors have nothing to disclose.
[a] Division of Cardiology, University of Minnesota Medical Center, 420 Delaware Street Southeast MMC 508, Minneapolis, MN 55455, USA; [b] Division of Cardiology, University of Washington Medical Center, 1959 NE Pacific St, Seattle, WA 98195, USA
* Corresponding author.
E-mail address: shkonety@umn.edu

Magn Reson Imaging Clin N Am 23 (2015) 105–116
http://dx.doi.org/10.1016/j.mric.2014.09.007
1064-9689/15/$ – see front matter © 2015 Elsevier Inc. All rights reserved.

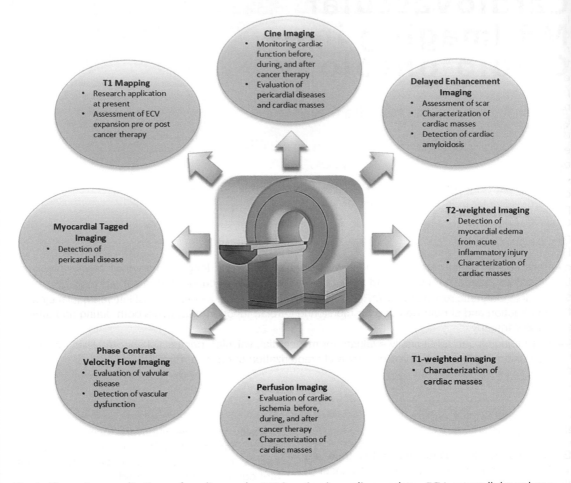

Fig. 1. The various applications of cardiovascular MR imaging in cardio-oncology. ECV, extracellular volume.

This article discusses the role of CMR imaging in the following 4 broad categories:

1. Cardiotoxicity of chemotherapeutic agents
2. Radiation-induced heart disease (RIHD)
3. Cardiac tumors
4. Other conditions pertinent to cardio-oncology

CARDIAC MAGNETIC RESONANCE IN THE DETECTION OF CARDIOTOXICITY FROM CHEMOTHERAPEUTIC AGENTS
Brief Overview of Cardiotoxicity

The occurrence of cardiotoxicity in the setting of chemotherapy can be variable and depends on the type of agent used, the overall cumulative dose administered, patient-related factors including age and comorbidities, as well as the use of adjunct therapies such as radiation.[5,7] Of the different classes of chemotherapeutic drugs that are implicated in causing cardiotoxicity, anthracyclines and tyrosine kinase inhibitor toxicities are well described.[7] In the case of anthracyclines, the incidence rates of acute, early-onset, and late-onset chronic progressive forms of cardiotoxicity are less than 1%, 1.6% to 2.1%, and 1.6% to 5% respectively.[7,8] Incidence rates of cardiomyopathy and congestive heart failure greater than 36% have also been reported in patients receiving anthracycline doses of more than 600 mg per meter square of body surface area.[9] In a clinical trial of women receiving trastuzumab, a monoclonal antibody–based tyrosine kinase inhibitor, for HER2-positive breast cancer, symptomatic congestive heart failure and asymptomatic 10% or more reduction in LVEF occurred in 1.7% and 7% of patients respectively.[10] The incidence of trastuzumab-induced cardiotoxicity is even higher in real-life settings than is observed in clinical trials.[11,12]

The pathophysiologic mechanisms underlying chemotherapy-induced cardiotoxicity are complex and incompletely understood. Anthracyclines are thought to promote formation of free radicals, leading to myocardial injury, whereas inhibition of cardiomyocyte human epidermal growth factor receptor-2 resulting in ATP depletion and contractile dysfunction contributes to the cardiotoxic effects of trastuzumab.[7] Despite deferring proposed pathophysiologic mechanisms, the end result ranges from clinically silent phenomena requiring coordinated surveillance through the use of biomarkers and cardiac imaging, to gross evidence of cardiac dysfunction with overt signs of heart failure.[13,14]

There is no universally accepted definition for chemotherapy-induced cardiotoxicity. A definition proposed by the Cardiac Review and Evaluation Committee supervising trastuzumab clinical trials relies on LVEF for identification of cardiac injury.[15] By this definition, cardiac toxicity from cancer chemotherapeutic agents refers to a decline in LVEF by 5% or more to less than 55% in the setting of heart failure, or an asymptomatic reduction in ejection fraction by at least 10%.[15] LVEF assessment by radionuclide imaging[16] and echocardiography[17] have been incorporated into clinical practice guidelines even though ejection fraction, by itself, may not be an accurate predictor of cardiotoxicity.[18] In addition, significant measurement variability, as well as issues with methodology, including image quality, geometric assumptions, and dependence on loading conditions, may limit detection of small but important changes when using LVEF measured by echocardiography.[19]

Detection of Early Cardiac Injury

CMR is considered to be the gold standard for the measurement of left ventricular volume, ejection fraction, and mass.[20–22] Based on limited evidence from small, mostly single-center studies, it may have the capability to detect subtle changes in left ventricular volume[23,24] and ejection fraction[23] and increase in myocardial mass in the acute stage of early anthracycline-induced injury, presumably from cardiac edema.[25] MR imaging also offers the unique advantage of characterizing tissues based on inherent differences in their magnetic properties (ie, T1, T2, and T2* relaxation times). In anthracycline-induced cardiotoxicity, there is potential expansion of extravascular space through myofibril loss, vacuolar degeneration, and inflammation.[9] CMR offers an opportunity to detect myocardial inflammation and edema during early stages of cardiac injury.[6,25] In a small, single-center study of 22 patients, early myocardial gadolinium enhancement on T1-weighted fast-spin echo imaging was linked to acute injury from anthracycline therapy and this

was associated with significant reduction in LVEF during the first month of treatment.[26] Early detection of myocardial edema by T2-weighted short-tau inversion recovery sequence, previously described as an indicator of acute injury in various disease processes,[27] was also shown to predict a reduction in LVEF at 1 year in a preliminary single-center study involving 28 patients with breast cancer who received anthracyclines.[25] Myocardial strain imaging is another promising CMR technique that can be used to assess early cardiac injury.[25] In a proof-of-concept study involving 10 patients with hematologic malignancy treated with a regimen containing anthracyclines, 3-month posttreatment global circumferential strain, but not global longitudinal strain, was significantly decreased compared with pretreatment values.[28] Note that data pertaining to the use of T1-weighted or T2-weighted imaging to evaluate early changes from cardiotoxicity, as well as strain imaging, are limited and require further studies to validate their clinical use for diagnostic or prognostic purposes.[6,25]

Detection of Late Cardiac Injury

Given the traditional reliance on reduced LVEF for the diagnosis of cardiotoxicity and the ability of CMR to accurately quantify LVEF, it may be used to identify patients who could be missed when conventional imaging methods are used. A higher prevalence of cardiomyopathy was detected by CMR in adult survivors of childhood cancers treated with anthracycline, compared with two-dimensional echocardiography.[29] CMR can also identify long-term cardiac sequelae of cancer chemotherapy such as left ventricular dysfunction,[29,30] reduced left ventricular mass index,[31] and right ventricular dysfunction.[30]

CMR is the imaging modality of choice to evaluate the presence of myocardial fibrosis, which is known to be a ubiquitous histopathologic feature of a broad variety of cardiomyopathies.[32] Distinct patterns of late gadolinium enhancement (LGE) are recognized on CMR correlating with a specific cause.[33] This is of particular importance during the assessment of chemotherapy induced cardiomyopathy, in individuals with preexisting cardiac conditions, such as, coronary artery disease (**Fig. 2**). The prevalence of LGE in cardiotoxicity is low.[25,31] Delayed enhancement patterns of the left ventricle seen on CMR include subepicardial LGE of the lateral,[34,35] inferolateral,[36] and septal[35] walls in trastuzumab-induced toxicity; and midmyocardial LGE of the inferolateral wall[28] and right ventricular insertion point[31] in anthracycline-induced toxicity.

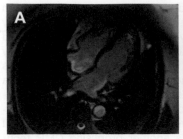
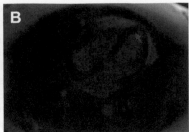
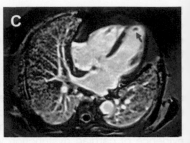

Fig. 2. Remote history of coronary artery disease in a patient with acute myelogenous leukemia. Four-chamber view of the heart using steady-state free precession cine imaging shows apical wall thinning and a hypointense mass in the left ventricular apex concerning for thrombus (*red arrow, A*). Inversion recovery imaging with a TI (inversion time) of 600 ms confirms the presence of an apical thrombus (*red arrow, B*). Delayed enhancement imaging additionally shows transmural late gadolinium enhancement of the anteroseptum and apex (*C*).

Although LGE is the gold standard to identify focal areas of myocardial fibrosis,[37] it is not well suited to assessing diffuse interstitial fibrosis, which is seen in cardiomyopathy caused by cardiotoxicity.[38,39] Techniques such as native T1 mapping and quantification of extracellular volume (ECV) fraction may better depict diffuse fibrosis,[40,41] and perhaps provide the ability to detect subclinical cardiac damage before decline in LVEF (**Fig. 3**). Evidence is now emerging for the prognostic significance of increased ECV fraction in predicting hard cardiovascular events, including all-cause mortality in broad populations.[42,43] However, robust data are lacking for its application in cardiotoxicity.

In 30 pediatric patients (mean age, 15.2 years) with normal LVEF and 2 years or more after anthracycline therapy, increased ECV correlated with surrogate end points such as decreased left ventricular mass and wall thickness, lower peak oxygen uptake on cardiopulmonary stress test, and higher anthracycline cumulative dose.[44] In another small single-center study of 42 adults (mean age, 55 years) who presented at a median time interval of 84 months following anthracycline therapy, diastolic dysfunction and increased left atrial volumes correlated with increased ECV.[45]

CARDIAC MAGNETIC RESONANCE IN RADIATION-INDUCED HEART DISEASE

Radiotherapy is an essential component of contemporary cancer treatment and it is estimated that external beam radiation is used at least once in 52% of all patients with cancer.[46] Inadvertent exposure of the heart to radiation during treatment of various malignancies involving the thorax and chest wall is considered to be the cause of RIHD.[47] The aggregate incidence of RIHD is estimated at 10% to 30% by 5 to 10 years after treatment and injury seems to be potentiated by the use of concurrent

chemotherapy.[48] RIHD is a major nonmalignant source of mortality among long-term cancer survivors who have received radiation.[48,49] Almost all cardiac structures are susceptible to radiation injury.[47,48,50,51] Although not common, damage from ionizing radiation can manifest early as acute myocarditis and pericarditis.[51] The late cardiovascular effects of radiation injury mostly include coronary artery disease (CAD) secondary to fibrointimal proliferation, classically affecting the ostia and proximal segments; myocardial fibrosis resulting in systolic and/or diastolic ventricular dysfunction; stenotic and regurgitant valvular heart lesions; conduction system disorders; and pericardial disease manifesting as chronic pericardial effusion or constrictive pericarditis.[48,51–53]

Given the wide spectrum of cardiac manifestations of RIHD, CMR offers a unique advantage to the clinician in being the comprehensive imaging modality. Cine imaging for cardiac anatomy and morphology, velocity-encoded or phase-contrast imaging for valvular function, T1 mapping/ECV quantification and LGE imaging for microscopic and macroscopic myocardial scar evaluation respectively, and stress perfusion imaging for the presence and extent of ischemia can provide valuable information in the clinical decision-making process.[53]

In long-term cancer survivors who have received radiotherapy, reversible perfusion defects are seen using single-photon emission tomography (SPECT).[54,55] Because of the strong association between RIHD and increased major cardiovascular events,[56–58] the high sensitivity and negative predictive value of stress MR imaging compared with SPECT in the evaluation of CAD[59] may have some utility.

A growing body of evidence supports the adverse prognostic implications of LGE in ischemic or nonischemic cardiomyopathies.[60–63] Even though fixed perfusion defects are found on

SPECT in individuals who have received medias-tinal radiation,[54,64,65] patterns of LGE and their prognostic implications need to be well defined in RIHD. LGE involving basal left ventricular seg-ments can be seen in RIHD.[66,67] Assessment of myocardial fibrosis by T1 mapping techniques is also potentially valuable in RIHD but their roles remain to be investigated.[53]

Another strength of CMR is in the evaluation of pericardial diseases, in which it offers integrated morphologic, functional, and physiologic data.[53,68] This strength can be especially useful in differentiating between constrictive pericarditis and restrictive cardiomyopathy, which may over-lap in RIHD.[69] The combination of features favor-ing constriction include increased pericardial thickness, systemic venous dilatation, inspiratory septal bounce indicating ventricular interdepen-dence, and tagged CMR depicting adhesions of pericardial layers.[68]

Despite the promise CMR possesses, hard trial evidence with respect to its use in the evaluation of RIHD is largely lacking. More studies are needed to accurately describe the prevalence, patterns, and prognostic significance of CMR find-ings in RIHD.

CARDIAC MAGNETIC RESONANCE IN THE ASSESSMENT OF CARDIAC MASSES

Tumors of the heart, whether primary or second-ary, are rare, with prevalence rates of 0.056% and 1.23%, respectively.[70] Clinical manifestations of cardiac tumors are varied. They range from be-ing incidental findings on imaging to causing constitutional symptoms and systemic embolic events, and because of their location they can pre-sent mimicking myocardial, valvular, or pericardial diseases.[71,72] Primary cardiac tumors are largely benign.[71] The most common are myxomas, fol-lowed by papillary fibroelastomas, fibromas, and lipomas.[73] Primary malignant tumors of the heart are extremely rare and most of them are sar-comas, followed by lymphoma.[73] Secondary or metastatic cardiac tumors have a 100 times higher incidence than primary neoplasms.[74] The com-mon sources are carcinomas of the lung, breast, esophagus; hematologic malignancies; and melanoma.[74]

In contrast with other imaging techniques, CMR offers unique advantages in the evaluation of car-diac masses.[75,76] Tumors generally contain larger cells and show more reactive inflammation

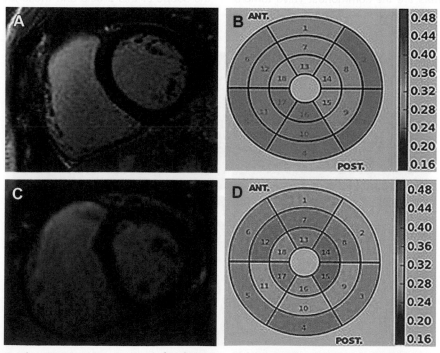

Fig. 3. Comparative CMR imaging methods for detection of a myocardial fibrosis in a healthy control (*A* and *C*) and an asymptomatic subject treated 5 years previously with anthracyclines (*B* and *D*). *A* and *B* shows standard LGE images for detection of replacement myocardial fibrosis and are both normal. *C* and *D* show in a color-coded bull's eye LV segmental format objective measurement of diffuse fibrosis and calculation of ECV. The normal control had an ECV of 0.27 (*C*, normal range 0.23-32). The patient with prior chemotherapy had an elevated ECV of 0.35 (*D*). (*Courtesy of* TG Neilan, Boston, MA.)

compared with normal tissue, and hence have higher free-water content and longer T1 and T2 relaxation times. This difference creates the inherent contrast that differentiates normal and neoplastic cells by MR imaging.[77,78] CMR gives accurate anatomic definition and tissue characterization using T1-weighted, T2-weighted, and gadolinium-enhanced sequences, whereas the functional impact of the mass can be assessed by cine imaging.[77,79] The malignant or benign nature of a cardiac mass can be assessed using CMR in many cases. Tumor size greater than 5 cm, infiltration of adjacent structures, and the presence of pericardial or pleural effusions are highly specific but less sensitive features of a malignant process, whereas location outside the left heart, tissue inhomogeneity, and contrast enhancement are highly sensitive but less specific features (**Fig. 4**).[80]

In addition to lack of the aforementioned features of malignancy, benign cardiac tumors originate from characteristic anatomic locations. Myxomas are typically located in the left atrium, attached to the interatrial septum via a thin stalk.[79] They are generally isointense on T1-weighted imaging, have higher signal intensity on T2-weighted images, and enhance heterogeneously with gadolinium.[77,79] Fibroelastomas are the commonest valve tumors and mostly occur on the aortic valve.[73] They are best diagnosed by echocardiography because of their small size and high mobility.[79] Fibromas are usually solitary intramural tumors. They are hypointense on both T1-weighted and T2-weighted imaging, lack contrast enhancement during first-pass perfusion imaging because of their avascularity, and characteristically show intense LGE.[79,81] Lipomas can occur in any cardiac chamber[71] and have homogeneous hyperintense signal on T1-weighted images that is markedly suppressed on fat-saturation imaging.

The MR imaging appearances of primary malignant tumors can overlap[77,79,81] and probably require tissue biopsy for confirmation. They share features characteristic of a malignant mass, as mentioned earlier. Metastatic cardiac tumors are diagnosed not only by their features on imaging but also from the knowledge of primary tumor elsewhere (**Fig. 5**).

CMR is also important in the depiction of cardiac masses that can masquerade as tumors. Prominent Coumadin ridge, lipomatous hypertrophy of the interatrial septum, thrombus, pericardial cysts, giant coronary aneurysms and so forth comprise the so-called pseudotumors and they are easily identifiable by CMR.[79] Comprehensive review of the CMR features of cardiac tumors is beyond the scope of this article and these are described elsewhere.[77,79]

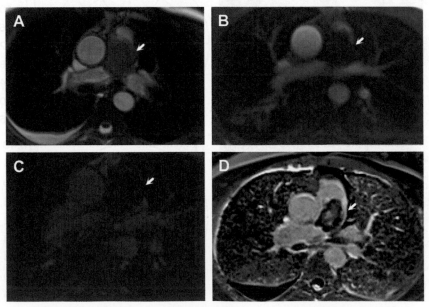

Fig. 4. Pulmonary artery sarcoma. Axial images of the main pulmonary artery (MPA) and mass (*arrows*) are shown at the level of the proximal ascending aorta. (*A*) A large mass almost obstructing the MPA on steady-state free precession cine imaging. There was subtle enhancement on first-pass perfusion imaging (*B*) and hypoenhancement on inversion recovery imaging with a TI of 600 milliseconds (*C*). On delayed gadolinium imaging (*D*) there was heterogenous enhancement favoring a tumor rather than a thrombus. The mass was subsequently proved to be a sarcoma by biopsy.

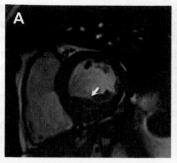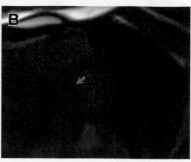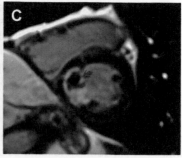

Fig. 5. Cardiac metastasis in a patient with renal cancer. Image *A* shows focal thickening in the basal inferior wall and infero-septum of the left ventricle (*white arrow*) acquired by steady-state free precession cine imaging in the short axis view. This area of thickening shows a core of hypoenhancement on inversion recovery imaging with a TI of 600 ms (*B, yellow arrow*). On delayed enhancement imaging, there is heterogeneous enhancement of the mass with a bright periphery and a central area of hypointensity, showing increased vascularity in the periphery and necrosis in the core (*C, red arrow*).

CARDIAC MAGNETIC RESONANCE IN OTHER CONDITIONS PERTINENT TO CARDIO-ONCOLOGY

Cardiac Magnetic Resonance in Vascular Injury Related to Cancer Therapy

Chemotherapeutic agents, such as tyrosine kinase inhibitors,[82] and androgen deprivation therapies[83] predispose individuals not only to cardiomyopathy but also to long-term cardiovascular events such as myocardial infarction and stroke. This predisposition can be partly explained by the presence of concurrent cardiovascular risk factors and effects of cancer therapy.[84] Endothelial dysfunction, which is pivotal in the development of atherosclerosis,[85] may also be important in the genesis of vascular disease. Patients treated with androgen deprivation therapy for prostate cancer have reduced brachial flow-mediated dilatation.[86] In experimental animal models, doxorubicin causes coronary arteriolar wall thickening[87] and endothelial dysfunction.[88]

Using phase-contrast MR (PC-MR) imaging, the vascular effect of chemotherapy was studied recently.[89] In this technique, a cross-sectional view of the aorta was acquired at the level of the main pulmonary artery. Aortic distensibility was calculated by dividing the change in aortic area in a cardiac cycle by the pulse pressure (measured by brachial blood pressure cuff at the time of PC-MR image acquisition), and multiplying it by the aortic area at end diastole. In this prospective study, aortic distensibility was measured on 53 individuals before and 4 months after anthracycline treatment. Patients treated with anthracycline had increased aortic stiffness (decreased distensibility) compared with pretreatment values, whereas that of healthy controls remained stable. This finding still applied even after adjusting for

age, sex, cardiac output, cardiac medications, and underlying clinical conditions like hypertension, which are known to influence aortic distensibility. Measurements of aortic stiffness may have clinical implications because it has been associated with reduced peak oxygen consumption and exercise intolerance.[90,91]

An additional role of CMR is imaging of aortic diseases for radiation-induced injury when clinically indicated. The aortic lumen, wall, and flow can be assessed without ionizing radiation, which is an advantage compared with computed tomography angiography.[53,75]

Cardiac Magnetic Resonance in Monitoring Response to Cardioprotective Therapy

In the past decade, some prospective clinical trials have evaluated the cardioprotective effect of β-blockers (BB),[92] angiotensin-converting enzyme inhibitors (ACEi),[93] or both[94] in patients undergoing intensive chemotherapy. The end points used in these trials were LVEF measured by echocardiography[92,93] or both echocardiography and CMR.[94] At present, PRADA (Prevention of Cardiac Dysfunction during an Adjuvant Breast Cancer Therapy)[95] and MANTICORE (Multidisciplinary Approach to Novel Therapies in Cardiology Oncology Research) 101-Breast[96] trials are underway to assess the efficacy of BB or ACEi therapy using CMR-based LVEF and left ventricular end-diastolic volume measurements as primary end points respectively.

Cardiac Magnetic Resonance in Amyloid Light Chain Amyloidosis

There are several types of amyloidoses[97]; of these, amyloid light-chain (AL) amyloidosis deserves a brief discussion in the context of cardio-oncology. AL amyloidosis is a plasma cell dyscrasia in which there is clonal production of immunoglobulin light chains with subsequent deposition in multiple organs.[98] The heart is involved about 50% of the time[99] and heart failure is the cause of death in most patients.[100]

Echocardiogram is the traditional noninvasive test of choice but has limitations.[101] The diagnosis of cardiac amyloidosis can be made accurately by CMR.[75,102] In addition to features that can also be seen by echocardiogram (ie, small left ventricle, biventricular hypertrophy, atrial septal thickening, biatrial enlargement, and restrictive filling pattern),[99,101] global subendocardial LGE and abnormal blood-myocardial gadolinium kinetics are characteristic CMR findings.[102] Abnormal blood-myocardial gadolinium kinetics refers to considerably reduced T1 relaxation time of the myocardium caused by retention of contrast in the expanded interstitium.[102,103] Thus, in patients suspected of having cardiac amyloidosis, demonstration of myocardial signal crossing the null point (becoming black) faster than or at the same time as the blood pool can be used as the basis for reliable visual assessment.[103] Pericardial and pleural effusions are other notable features in cardiac amyloidosis.[104]

SUMMARY

In the current era of multimodality imaging, CMR provides unique advantages compared with other imaging modalities in cardio-oncology. Its unsurpassed accuracy in the measurement of cardiac volume and its derivative ejection fraction can be used for conventional surveillance and monitoring of patients before and after chemotherapy as recommended by oncologic guidelines. The ability to assess myocardial inflammation, edema, and fibrosis enables clinicians to identify patients with both early and late stages of radiation or chemotherapy-induced cardiac injury. Newer techniques such as T1 mapping and ECV fraction estimation, which have enabled imaging of the interstitium, seem highly promising in the early detection of cardiotoxicity. Imaging of the vasculature, cardiac tumors, and other oncologic entities such as amyloidosis have now become mainstream applications of CMR. In our experience, the most common indication for CMR in cardio-oncology patients is to assess LVEF before and during chemotherapy. A stress MR is often recommended in patients with multiple cardiac risk factors or if there are ECG abnormalities at baseline, prior to stem cell transplantation or initiation of chemotherapy with known cardiotoxicity, to exclude subclinical coronary artery disease. CMR is ideal to establish a good baseline assessment of LV function and viability in patients with known coronary artery disease prior to advanced cancer therapies such as stem cell transplantation. Given the depth of information that can be obtained by CMR, it is well poised to be the preferred imaging modality in cardio-oncology.

REFERENCES

1. American Cancer Society. Cancer facts & figure 2014. Available at: http://www.cancer.org/acs/groups/content/@research/documents/webcontent/acspc-042151.pdf. Accessed May 29, 2014.
2. Yeh ET, Tong AT, Lenihan DJ, et al. Cardiovascular complications of cancer therapy: diagnosis, pathogenesis, and management. Circulation 2004; 109(25):3122–31.
3. Patnaik JL, Byers T, DiGuiseppi C, et al. Cardiovascular disease competes with breast cancer as the leading cause of death for older females diagnosed with breast cancer: a retrospective cohort study. Breast Cancer Res 2011;13(3):R64.
4. Shenoy C, Klem I, Crowley AL, et al. Cardiovascular complications of breast cancer therapy in older adults. Oncologist 2011;16(8):1138–43.
5. Bovelli D, Plataniotis G, Roila F. Cardiotoxicity of chemotherapeutic agents and radiotherapy-related heart disease: ESMO clinical practice guidelines. Ann Oncol 2010;21(Suppl 5):v277–82.
6. Vasu S, Hundley WG. Understanding cardiovascular injury after treatment for cancer: an overview of current uses and future directions of cardiovascular magnetic resonance. J Cardiovasc Magn Reson 2013;15(1):66.
7. Yeh ET, Bickford CL. Cardiovascular complications of cancer therapy: incidence, pathogenesis, diagnosis, and management. J Am Coll Cardiol 2009; 53(24):2231–47.
8. Wouters KA, Kremer LC, Miller TL, et al. Protecting against anthracycline-induced myocardial damage: a review of the most promising strategies. Br J Haematol 2005;131(5):561–78.
9. Singal PK, Iliskovic N. Doxorubicin-induced cardiomyopathy. N Engl J Med 1998;339:900–5.
10. Untch M, Smith I, Gianni L, et al. Trastuzumab after adjuvant chemotherapy in HER2-positive breast cancer. N Engl J Med 2005;353:1659–72.
11. Vaz-Luis I, Keating NL, Lin NU, et al. Duration and toxicity of adjuvant trastuzumab in older patients with early-stage breast cancer: a population-based study. J Clin Oncol 2014;32(9):927–34.
12. Chen J, Long JB, Hurria A, et al. Incidence of heart failure or cardiomyopathy after adjuvant trastuzumab therapy for breast cancer. J Am Coll Cardiol 2012;60(24):2504–12.

13. Jurcut R, Wildiers H, Ganame J, et al. Detection and monitoring of cardiotoxicity-what does modern cardiology offer? Support Care Cancer 2008;16(5):437–45.

14. Kerkhove D, Fontaine C, Droogmans S, et al. How to monitor cardiac toxicity of chemotherapy: time is muscle. Heart 2013;100(15):1208–17.

15. Seidman A, Hudis C, Pierri MK, et al. Cardiac dysfunction in the trastuzumab clinical trials experience. J Clin Oncol 2002;20(5):1215–21.

16. Klocke FJ, Baird MG, Bateman TM, et al. ACC/AHA guideline ACC/AHA/ASNC guidelines for the clinical use of cardiac radionuclide imaging — executive summary: a report of the American College of Cardiology/American Heart Association Task Force on practice guidelines (ACC/AHA/ASNC Committee to Revise the 1995 Guidelines for the Clinical Use of Radionuclide Imaging). J Am Coll Cardiol 2003;42:1318–33.

17. Cheitlin MD, Armstrong WF, Aurigemma GP, et al. ACC/AHA/ASE 2003 guideline update for the clinical application of echocardiography: summary article: a report of the American College of Cardiology/American Heart Association Task Force on Practice Guidelines (ACC/AHA/ASE Committee to Update the 1997 Guidelines for the Clinical Application of Echocardiography). Circulation 2003; 108(9):1146–62.

18. Swain SM, Whaley FS, Ewer MS. Congestive heart failure in patients treated with doxorubicin: a retrospective analysis of three trials. Cancer 2003; 97(11):2869–79.

19. Oreto L, Todaro MC, Umland MM, et al. Use of echocardiography to evaluate the cardiac effects of therapies used in cancer treatment: what do we know? J Am Soc Echocardiogr 2012;25(11):1141–52.

20. Pennell DJ, Sechtem UP, Higgins CB, et al. Clinical indications for cardiovascular magnetic resonance (CMR): Consensus Panel report. Eur Heart J 2004; 25(21):1940–65.

21. Pennell DJ. Ventricular volume and mass by CMR. J Cardiovasc Magn Reson 2003;4(4):507–13.

22. Pennell DJ. Cardiovascular magnetic resonance. Circulation 2010;121(5):692–705.

23. Drafts BC, Twomley KM, D'Agostino R, et al. Low to moderate dose anthracycline-based chemotherapy is associated with early noninvasive imaging evidence of subclinical cardiovascular disease. JACC Cardiovasc Imaging 2013;6(8):877–85.

24. Grover S, DePasquale C, Leong DP, et al. Early cardiac changes following anthracycline chemotherapy in breast cancer: a prospective multicentre study using advanced cardiac imaging and biochemical markers. J Cardiovasc Magn Reson 2012;14(Suppl 1):P181.

25. Thavendiranathan P, Wintersperger BJ, Flamm SD, et al. Cardiac MRI in the assessment of cardiac injury and toxicity from cancer chemotherapy: a systematic review. Circ Cardiovasc Imaging 2013; 6(6):1080–91.

26. Wassmuth R, Lentzsch S, Erdbruegger U, et al. Subclinical cardiotoxic effects of anthracyclines as assessed by magnetic resonance imaging-a pilot study. Am Heart J 2001;141(6):1007–13.

27. Francone M, Carbone I, Agati L, et al. Utility of T2-weighted short-tau inversion recovery (STIR) sequences in cardiac MRI: an overview of clinical applications in ischaemic and non-ischaemic heart disease. Radiol Med 2011;116(1):32–46.

28. Lunning MA, Kutty S, Rome ET, et al. Cardiac magnetic resonance imaging for the assessment of the myocardium after doxorubicin-based chemotherapy. Am J Clin Oncol 2013. [Epub ahead of print].

29. Armstrong GT, Plana JC, Zhang N, et al. Screening adult survivors of childhood cancer for cardiomyopathy: comparison of echocardiography and cardiac magnetic resonance imaging. J Clin Oncol 2012;30(23):2876–84.

30. Ylänen K, Poutanen T, Savikurki-Heikkilä P, et al. Cardiac magnetic resonance imaging in the evaluation of the late effects of anthracyclines among long-term survivors of childhood cancer. J Am Coll Cardiol 2013;61(14):1539–47.

31. Neilan TG, Coelho-Filho OR, Pena-Herrera D, et al. Left ventricular mass in patients with a cardiomyopathy after treatment with anthracyclines. Am J Cardiol 2012;110(11):1679–86.

32. Mewton N, Liu CY, Croisille P, et al. Assessment of myocardial fibrosis with cardiovascular magnetic resonance. J Am Coll Cardiol 2011;57(8):891–903.

33. Senthilkumar A, Majmudar MD, Shenoy C, et al. Identifying the etiology: a systematic approach using delayed-enhancement cardiovascular magnetic resonance. Heart Fail Clin 2009;5(3):349–67.

34. Wadhwa D, Fallah-Rad N, Grenier D, et al. Trastuzumab mediated cardiotoxicity in the setting of adjuvant chemotherapy for breast cancer: a retrospective study. Breast Cancer Res Treat 2009; 117(2):357–64.

35. Fallah-Rad N, Lytwyn M, Fang T, et al. Delayed contrast enhancement cardiac magnetic resonance imaging in trastuzumab induced cardiomyopathy. J Cardiovasc Magn Reson 2008;10:5.

36. Lawley C, Wainwright C, Segelov E, et al. Pilot study evaluating the role of cardiac magnetic resonance imaging in monitoring adjuvant trastuzumab therapy for breast cancer. Asia Pac J Clin Oncol 2012;8(1):95–100.

37. Wagner A, Mahrholdt H, Holly TA, et al. Contrast-enhanced MRI and routine single photon emission computed tomography (SPECT) perfusion imaging for detection of subendocardial myocardial infarcts: an imaging study. Lancet 2003;361(9355): 374–9.

38. Bernaba BN, Chan JB, Lai CK, et al. Pathology of late-onset anthracycline cardiomyopathy. Cardiovasc Pathol 2010;19(5):308–11.

39. Ugander M, Oki AJ, Hsu L-Y, et al. Extracellular volume imaging by magnetic resonance imaging provides insights into overt and sub-clinical myocardial pathology. Eur Heart J 2012;33(10):1268–78.

40. Moon JC, Messroghli DR, Kellman P, et al. Myocardial T1 mapping and extracellular volume quantification: a Society for Cardiovascular Magnetic Resonance (SCMR) and CMR Working Group of the European Society of Cardiology consensus statement. J Cardiovasc Magn Reson 2013; 15(1):92.

41. Salerno M, Kramer CM. Advances in parametric mapping with CMR imaging. JACC Cardiovasc Imaging 2013;6(7):806–22.

42. Wong TC, Piehler KM, Kang IA, et al. Myocardial extracellular volume fraction quantified by cardiovascular magnetic resonance is increased in diabetes and associated with mortality and incident heart failure admission. Eur Heart J 2014;35(10): 657–64.

43. Wong TC, Piehler K, Meier CG, et al. Association between extracellular matrix expansion quantified by cardiovascular magnetic resonance and short-term mortality. Circulation 2012;126(10): 1206–16.

44. Tham EB, Haykowsky MJ, Chow K, et al. Diffuse myocardial fibrosis by T1-mapping in children with subclinical anthracycline cardiotoxicity: relationship to exercise capacity, cumulative dose and remodeling. J Cardiovasc Magn Reson 2013; 15(1):48.

45. Neilan TG, Coelho-Filho OR, Shah RV, et al. Myocardial extracellular volume by cardiac magnetic resonance imaging in patients treated with anthracycline-based chemotherapy. Am J Cardiol 2013;111(5):717–22.

46. Delaney G, Jacob S, Featherstone C, et al. The role of radiotherapy in cancer treatment: estimating optimal utilization from a review of evidence-based clinical guidelines. Cancer 2005;104(6): 1129–37.

47. Darby SC, Cutter DJ, Boerma M, et al. Radiation-related heart disease: current knowledge and future prospects. Int J Radiat Oncol Biol Phys 2010;76(3):656–65.

48. Carver JR, Shapiro CL, Ng A, et al. American Society of Clinical Oncology clinical evidence review on the ongoing care of adult cancer survivors: cardiac and pulmonary late effects. J Clin Oncol 2007; 25(25):3991–4008.

49. Aleman BM, van den Belt-Dusebout AW, Klokman WJ, et al. Long-term cause-specific mortality of patients treated for Hodgkin's disease. J Clin Oncol 2003;21(18):3431–9.

50. Veinot JP, Edwards WD. Pathology of radiation-induced heart disease: a surgical and autopsy study of 27 cases. Hum Pathol 1996;27(8):766–73.

51. Heidenreich PA, Kapoor JR. Radiation induced heart disease: systemic disorders in heart disease. Heart 2009;95(3):252–8.

52. Yusuf SW, Sami S, Daher IN. Radiation-induced heart disease: a clinical update. Cardiol Res Pract 2011;2011:317659.

53. Lancellotti P, Nkomo VT, Badano LP, et al. Expert consensus for multi-modality imaging evaluation of cardiovascular complications of radiotherapy in adults: a report from the European Association of Cardiovascular Imaging and the American Society of Echocardiography. Eur Heart J Cardiovasc Imaging 2013;14(8):721–40.

54. Seddon B, Cook A, Gothard L, et al. Detection of defects in myocardial perfusion imaging in patients with early breast cancer treated with radiotherapy. Radiother Oncol 2002;64(1):53–63.

55. Correa CR, Litt HI, Hwang WT, et al. Coronary artery findings after left-sided compared with right-sided radiation treatment for early-stage breast cancer. J Clin Oncol 2007;25(21):3031–7.

56. Darby SC, Ewertz M, McGale P, et al. Risk of ischemic heart disease in women after radiotherapy for breast cancer. N Engl J Med 2013; 368(11):987–98.

57. Shimizu Y, Kodama K, Nishi N, et al. Radiation exposure and circulatory disease risk: Hiroshima and Nagasaki atomic bomb survivor data, 1950-2003. BMJ 2010;340:b5349.

58. Carr ZA, Land CE, Kleinerman RA, et al. Coronary heart disease after radiotherapy for peptic ulcer disease. Int J Radiat Oncol Biol Phys 2005;61(3): 842–50.

59. Greenwood JP, Maredia N, Younger JF, et al. Cardiovascular magnetic resonance and single-photon emission computed tomography for diagnosis of coronary heart disease (CE-MARC): a prospective trial. Lancet 2012;379(9814):453–60.

60. Gao P, Yee R, Gula L, et al. Prediction of arrhythmic events in ischemic and dilated cardiomyopathy patients referred for implantable cardiac defibrillator: evaluation of multiple scar quantification measures for late gadolinium enhancement magnetic resonance imaging. Circ Cardiovasc Imaging 2012; 5(4):448–56.

61. Gulati A, Jabbour A, Ismail TF, et al. Association of fibrosis with mortality and sudden cardiac death in patients with nonischemic dilated cardiomyopathy. JAMA 2013;309(9):896–908.

62. Wu KC, Gerstenblith G, Guallar E, et al. Combined cardiac magnetic resonance imaging and C-reactive protein levels identify a cohort at low risk for defibrillator firings and death. Circ Cardiovasc Imaging 2012;5(2):178–86.

63. Klem I, Weinsaft JW, Bahnson TD, et al. Assessment of myocardial scarring improves risk stratification in patients evaluated for cardiac defibrillator implantation. J Am Coll Cardiol 2012; 60(5):408–20.

64. Prosnitz RG, Hubbs JL, Evans ES, et al. Prospective assessment of radiotherapy-associated cardiac toxicity in breast cancer patients: analysis of data 3 to 6 years after treatment. Cancer 2007; 110(8):1840–50.

65. Hardenbergh PH, Munley MT, Bentel GC, et al. Cardiac perfusion changes in patients treated for breast cancer with radiation therapy and doxorubicin: preliminary results. Int J Radiat Oncol Biol Phys 2001;49(4):1023–8.

66. O H-Icí D, Garot J. Radiation-induced heart disease. Circ Heart Fail 2011;4(1):e1–2.

67. Domoto S, Niinami H, Kimura F, et al. Clinical images of radiation-induced heart disease. Eur Heart J 2014;35(32):2196.

68. Bogaert J, Francone M. Cardiovascular magnetic resonance in pericardial diseases. J Cardiovasc Magn Reson 2009;11:14.

69. Yamada H, Tabata T, Jaffer SJ, et al. Clinical features of mixed physiology of constriction and restriction: echocardiographic characteristics and clinical outcome. Eur J Echocardiogr 2007;8(3): 185–94.

70. Lam KY, Dickens P, Chan AC. Tumors of the heart. A 20-year experience with a review of 12,485 consecutive autopsies. Arch Pathol Lab Med 1993;117(10):1027–31.

71. Bruce CJ. Cardiac tumours: diagnosis and management. Heart 2011;97(2):151–60.

72. Shapiro L. Cardiac tumours: diagnosis and management. Heart 2001;85(2):218–22.

73. Elbardissi AW, Dearani JA, Daly RC, et al. Survival after resection of primary cardiac tumors: a 48-year experience. Circulation 2008;118(14 Suppl):S7–15.

74. Reynen K. Metastases to the heart. Ann Oncol 2004;15(3):375–81.

75. Hundley WG, Bluemke DA, Finn JP, et al. ACCF/ ACR/AHA/NASCI/SCMR 2010 expert consensus document on cardiovascular magnetic resonance: a report of the American College of Cardiology Foundation Task Force on Expert Consensus Documents. J Am Coll Cardiol 2010;55(23):2614–62.

76. Grizzard JD, Ang GB. Magnetic resonance imaging of pericardial disease and cardiac masses. Cardiol Clin 2007;25(1):111–40, vi.

77. Sparrow PJ, Kurian JB, Jones TR. MR imaging of cardiac tumors. Radiographics 2005;25(5):1255–76.

78. Mitchell DG, Lawrence D. The biophysical basis of tissue contrast in extracranial MR imaging. AJR Am J Roentgenol 1987;149(4):831–7.

79. Motwani M, Kidambi A, Herzog BA, et al. MR imaging of cardiac tumors and masses: a review of methods and clinical applications. Radiology 2013;268(1):26–43.

80. Hoffmann U, Globits S, Schima W, et al. Usefulness of magnetic resonance imaging of cardiac and paracardiac masses. Am J Cardiol 2003;92(7):890–5.

81. O'Donnell DH, Abbara S, Chaithiraphan V, et al. Cardiac tumors: optimal cardiac MR sequences and spectrum of imaging appearances. AJR Am J Roentgenol 2009;193(2):377–87.

82. Chu TF, Rupnick MA, Kerkela R, et al. Cardiotoxicity associated with tyrosine kinase inhibitor sunitinib. Lancet 2007;370(9604):2011–9.

83. Saigal CS, Gore JL, Krupski TL, et al. Androgen deprivation therapy increases cardiovascular morbidity in men with prostate cancer. Cancer 2007;110(7):1493–500.

84. Meacham LR, Chow EJ, Ness KK, et al. Cardiovascular risk factors in adult survivors of pediatric cancer–a report from the childhood cancer survivor study. Cancer Epidemiol Biomarkers Prev 2010; 19(1):170–81.

85. Quyyumi AA. Endothelial function in health and disease: new insights into the genesis of cardiovascular disease. Am J Med 1998;105(1A):32S–9S.

86. Gilbert SE, Tew GA, Bourke L, et al. Assessment of endothelial dysfunction by flow-mediated dilatation in men on long-term androgen deprivation therapy for prostate cancer. Exp Physiol 2013; 98(9):1401–10.

87. Eckman DM, Stacey RB, Rowe R, et al. Weekly doxorubicin increases coronary arteriolar wall and adventitial thickness. PLoS One 2013;8(2):e57554.

88. Wolf MB, Baynes JW. The anti-cancer drug, doxorubicin, causes oxidant stress-induced endothelial dysfunction. Biochim Biophys Acta 2006;1760(2): 267–71.

89. Chaosuwannakit N, D'Agostino R, Hamilton CA, et al. Aortic stiffness increases upon receipt of anthracycline chemotherapy. J Clin Oncol 2010;28(1): 166–72.

90. Hundley WG, Kitzman DW, Morgan TM, et al. Cardiac cycle-dependent changes in aortic area and distensibility are reduced in older patients with isolated diastolic heart failure and correlate with exercise intolerance. J Am Coll Cardiol 2001; 38(3):796–802.

91. Rerkpattanapipat P, Hundley WG, Link KM, et al. Relation of aortic distensibility determined by magnetic resonance imaging in patients > or =60 years of age to systolic heart failure and exercise capacity. Am J Cardiol 2002;90(11):1221–5.

92. Kalay N, Basar E, Ozdogru I, et al. Protective effects of carvedilol against anthracycline-induced cardiomyopathy. J Am Coll Cardiol 2006;48(11): 2258–62.

93. Cardinale D, Colombo A, Sandri MT, et al. Prevention of high-dose chemotherapy-induced

cardiotoxicity in high-risk patients by angiotensin-converting enzyme inhibition. Circulation 2006; 114(23):2474–81.

94. Bosch X, Rovira M, Sitges M, et al. Enalapril and carvedilol for preventing chemotherapy-induced left ventricular systolic dysfunction in patients with malignant hemopathies: the OVERCOME trial (preventiOn of left Ventricular dysfunction with Enalapril and caRvedilol in patients submitted to intensive ChemOtherapy for the treatment of Malignant hEmopathies). J Am Coll Cardiol 2013; 61(23):2355–62.

95. Heck SL, Gulati G, Ree AH, et al. Rationale and design of the prevention of cardiac dysfunction during an adjuvant breast cancer therapy (PRADA) trial. Cardiology 2012;123(4):240–7.

96. Pituskin E, Haykowsky M, Mackey JR, et al. Rationale and design of the multidisciplinary approach to novel therapies in cardiology oncology research trial (MANTICORE 101–breast): a randomized, placebo-controlled trial to determine if conventional heart failure pharmacotherapy can prevent trastuzumab-mediated left ventricular remodeling among patients with HER2+ early breast cancer using cardiac MRI. BMC Cancer 2011;11(1):318.

97. Westermark P, Benson MD, Buxbaum JN, et al. A primer of amyloid nomenclature. Amyloid 2007; 14(3):179–83.

98. Merlini G, Wechalekar AD, Palladini G. Systemic light chain amyloidosis: an update for treating physicians. Blood 2013;121(26):5124–30.

99. Falk RH, Dubrey SW. Amyloid heart disease. Prog Cardiovasc Dis 2010;52(4):347–61.

100. Gertz MA, Rajkumar SV. Primary systemic amyloidosis. Curr Treat Options Oncol 2002;3(3):261–71.

101. Rahman JE, Helou EF, Gelzer-Bell R, et al. Noninvasive diagnosis of biopsy-proven cardiac amyloidosis. J Am Coll Cardiol 2004;43(3):410–5.

102. Maceira AM, Joshi J, Prasad SK, et al. Cardiovascular magnetic resonance in cardiac amyloidosis. Circulation 2005;111(2):186–93.

103. White JA, Kim HW, Shah D, et al. CMR imaging with rapid visual T1 assessment predicts mortality in patients suspected of cardiac amyloidosis. JACC Cardiovasc Imaging 2014;7(2):143–56.

104. Bogaert J, Taylor AM. Infiltrative and storage disease. In: Bogaert J, Dymarkowski S, Taylor AM, et al, editors. Clinical cardiac MRI. Heidelberg (Germany), New York, Dordrecht (Netherlands), London: Springer; 2012. p. 323–5.

Coronary MR Angiography Revealed
How to Optimize Image Quality

Masaki Ishida, MD, Hajime Sakuma, MD*

KEYWORDS

- Magnetic resonance imaging • Coronary magnetic resonance angiography
- Coronary artery disease • Respiratory gating • Cardiac gating • Gadolinium contrast medium

KEY POINTS

- Coronary magnetic resonance (MR) angiography permits noninvasive assessment of coronary artery disease without exposing patients to radiation or administration of contrast medium.
- Slower acquisition of coronary MR angiography necessitates the use of free-breathing, navigator echo respiratory gating acquisition to obtain coronary angiograms with high spatial resolution and full 3-dimensional coverage of the coronary artery tree.
- Use of an abdominal belt can reduce blurring and artifacts caused by respiratory motion on coronary MR angiography.
- Electrocardiographic acquisition with a narrow data-acquisition window (<50 milliseconds) in the cardiac cycle is important to reduce motion blurring of the coronary MR angiogram.
- A high parallel imaging factor achieved by 32-channel cardiac coils is of value to reduce overall imaging time and to shorten the data-acquisition window in the cardiac cycle.
- Steady-state free-precession sequences provide excellent blood contrast at 1.5 T without injection of contrast medium, whereas gradient-echo sequences are preferred at 3 T and higher field strengths.

INTRODUCTION

Coronary artery disease (CAD) is the leading cause of death in industrialized countries.[1] A large number of single-center and multicenter studies demonstrated high negative predictive value of coronary computed tomography (CT) angiography for ruling out obstructive CAD.[2] Although radiation exposure of multidetector-row CT (MDCT) has been steadily decreasing over the past decade, the radiation dose of coronary CT angiography with ordinary 64-slice MDCT is not negligible. In addition, the diagnostic accuracy of coronary CT angiography is reduced in patients with heavily calcified plaques in the coronary arterial wall. For the past 2 decades, a variety of MR imaging sequences and postprocessing techniques have been developed to make coronary MR angiography a noninvasive alternative to X-ray coronary angiography. Coronary MR angiography allows for visualization of luminal narrowing of the coronary artery without exposing patients to radiation or administration of contrast medium.[3–7] In addition, coronary MR angiography readily delineates the coronary arterial lumen in patients with heavily calcified plaques (**Fig. 1**). By using improved

The authors have nothing to disclose.
Department of Radiology, Mie University Hospital, 2-174 Edobashi, Tsu, Mie 514-8507, Japan
* Corresponding author.
E-mail address: sakuma@clin.medic.mie-u.ac.jp

Magn Reson Imaging Clin N Am 23 (2015) 117–125
http://dx.doi.org/10.1016/j.mric.2014.09.008
1064-9689/15/$ – see front matter

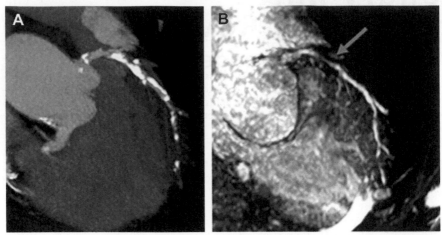

Fig. 1. In this 70-year-old man with chest exertion on effort, coronary computed tomography (CT) angiography (*A*) demonstrated that the proximal to mid left anterior descending artery (LAD) has severe calcification. In the coronary segment with severe calcification, it is impossible to judge if there is significant stenosis or not. On a whole-heart coronary MR angiogram (*B*), however, no significant stenosis was shown in the LAD where severe calcification was observed on the coronary CT angiography image (*arrow*). No significant stenosis was observed in invasive coronary angiography (not shown).

acquisition techniques such as high-field MR, 32-channel coils, and high parallel imaging factors, the image quality, diagnostic accuracy, imaging time, and study success rate of coronary MR angiography has steadily improved. Despite the recent progress in coronary MR angiography, its accessibility and effectiveness in patients with known or suspected CAD are still limited in comparison with stress perfusion MR imaging and late gadolinium-enhanced MR imaging.[8,9] This fact may be attributable to the complexity and operator dependency in setting up patients and choosing optimal acquisition parameters for coronary MR angiography. Consequently, this review describes how to optimize the image quality of coronary MR angiography regarding the aspects of respiratory gating and motion compensation, electrocardiography (ECG) gating, image-acquisition sequences, and preparation pulses.

IMAGING STRATEGIES FOR CORONARY MAGNETIC RESONANCE ANGIOGRAPHY

Coronary MR angiography is technically demanding because of the small size and tortuous course of the coronary artery. In addition, the complex motion caused by cardiac and respiratory motion poses a major challenge to coronary MR angiography. Therefore, high spatial resolution, volume coverage for the entire heart, and high contrast between coronary arterial lumen and the surrounding tissue are required for adequate visualization of the coronary artery vasculature.

Although breath-hold 3-dimensional (3D) coronary MR angiography has advantages in terms of time efficiency compared with free-breathing 3D coronary MR angiography, short imaging time is achieved at the expense of spatial resolution and volume coverage. Because of the considerably slower acquisition speed of MR angiography in comparison with MDCT, free-breathing coronary MR angiography using navigator echo respiratory gating has been a method of choice to achieve sufficient spatial resolution and volumetric coverage.[10–13] Today free-breathing 3D whole-heart coronary MR angiography is widely used for MR imaging of the coronary arteries because this approach has advantages, including:

- High signal-to-noise ratio (SNR)
- Sufficient spatial resolution for the detection of obstructive CAD
- Volumetric coverage of the entire coronary artery tree for a single 3D acquisition

The image quality of 3D whole-heart coronary MR angiography is determined by many factors, including:

- Respiratory gating and motion correction
- ECG gating
- Acquisition pulse sequence
- Preparation pulses such as fat suppression and T2 preparation

Magnetic field strength and administration of gadolinium-based contrast media also substantially influence image contrast on coronary MR angiography.

Respiratory Gating and Motion Compensation

Respiratory motion displaces the heart more than 2 cm, requiring the technique of respiratory motion compensation. The navigator technique uses a selective radiofrequency "pencil-beam" excitation to monitor the diaphragmatic position, usually on the dome of the right hemidiaphragm (**Fig. 2**). If the position of the lung-diaphragm interface is within a predefined acceptance window (typically ±2.5 mm) at the end-expiratory position, image data are accepted. Otherwise, image data are rejected and the data have to be remeasured in the next cardiac cycle. In this case coronary MR angiography data acquisition is continued until all necessary data in k-space are completed. The positional information of the lung-diaphragm interface by the navigator is also used for adoptive motion correction that can compensate the displacement of the coronary arteries by respiration for each acquisition.

Reduction of the acceptance window reduces the motion blurring but increases the overall acquisition time because more data are rejected. The major drawback of navigator echo free-breathing 3D whole-heart coronary MR angiography is its long acquisition time. This problem results in an increased susceptibility to motion problems (eg, drift of the diaphragm position, irregular breathing pattern, or heart rate variations during imaging). In early studies, the success rate of whole-heart coronary MR angiography remained in a range between 86% and 91%.[4–6]

To overcome this problem, several approaches have been proposed. First, the use of 32-channel cardiac coils and a higher parallel imaging factor has been proposed.[7] In a recent study by Nagata and colleagues,[7] the mean imaging time of whole-heart coronary MR angiography was significantly reduced from 12.3 ± 4.2 minutes with 5-channel coils to 6.3 ± 2.2 minutes using 32-channel coils. The reduction of imaging time leads to an improved study success rate (100%) without noticeable worsening of image quality.[7] Second, the abdominal belt helps to shorten the imaging time of whole-heart coronary MR angiography because it reduces the amplitude of diaphragmatic position and improves scan efficiency (**Fig. 3**).[14] A recent study by Ishida and colleagues[14] showed that application of the abdominal belt significantly improved scan efficiency and image quality of navigator-gated whole-heart coronary MR angiography in both United Kingdom and Japanese patient populations. With the combined use of 32-channel coils and the abdominal belt, the vessel-based sensitivity and specificity of 1.5-T whole-heart coronary MR angiography in

A

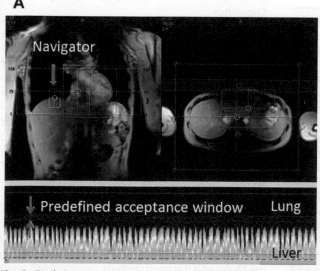

B

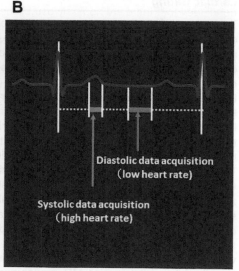

Fig. 2. Real-time prospective navigator echo technique. "Pencil-beam" navigator is positioned on the dome of right hemidiaphragm on coronary scout image. The upward and downward motion of the lung and diaphragm interface is shown as red dots along the bottom (*A*). Depending on the diaphragmatic position, the data are either accepted when the diaphragmatic position is within a predefined acceptance window, or rejected (*B*). In the latter case, the data have to be remeasured. Reduction of the acceptance window reduces the motion artifacts but increases the overall acquisition time because more data are rejected.

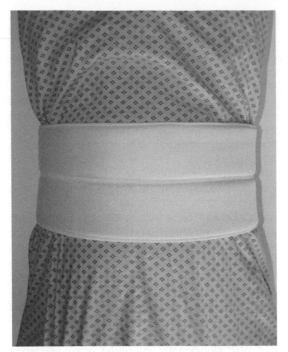

Fig. 3. The 20-cm wide abdominal belt was wrapped tightly around the patient's abdomen during end-expiration to suppress diaphragmatic motion.

the detection of significant stenosis reached 86% and 93%, respectively (**Fig. 4**).[7]

Cardiac Gating

To freeze the motion of the coronary artery by cardiac contraction and diastolic relaxation, data acquisition has to be synchronized to the cardiac cycle and to be adjusted to the periods with minimal motion of coronary arteries by using ECG gating.[15] The optimal delay time after ECG R wave and the length of the acquisition window in the cardiac cycle that can minimize blurring of the coronary artery depends not only on patients' heart rate but also other hemodynamic factors. Therefore, both trigger delay time and acquisition window in the cardiac cycle should be optimized in each patient.[15] To determine the subject-specific data-acquisition window in the cardiac cycle, cine MR images of high temporal resolution are acquired.[16] A trigger delay time and an interval of minimal motion of the coronary artery are visually determined on cine MR images acquired shortly before the coronary MR angiography, typically by referring the right coronary artery. Coronary MR angiography can be acquired in end-systole or during diastole, which has its own advantages and disadvantages (**Table 1**).

Free-breathing acquisition with the navigator echo technique allows for the use of narrow acquisition windows in the cardiac cycle that can effectively reduce motion blurring of the coronary artery. However, as the acquisition window is shortened, the overall scan time is prolonged. Higher parallel imaging factor achieved by 32-channel cardiac coils can reduce overall data-acquisition time of coronary MR angiography, which can be used not only to reduce total study time but also to narrow the acquisition window in the cardiac cycle without extending the scan time. In a study by Nagata and colleagues,[7] the mean acquisition window in the cardiac cycle using 32-channel cardiac coils and parallel imaging factor of 4 (84 ± 57 milliseconds for diastolic acquisition and 48 ± 18 milliseconds for systolic acquisition) was approximately half of that in a previous study using 5-channel cardiac coils (152 ± 67 milliseconds for diastolic acquisition and 98 ± 26 milliseconds for systolic acquisition) while the success rate, image quality, and overall scan time was comparable or slightly improved.[6] In patients with a high heart rate, a narrow acquisition window in the cardiac cycle (<50 milliseconds) is critically important for reducing motion blurring of the coronary artery on whole-heart coronary MR angiography. It should be noted that even in patients with a low heart rate, a narrow acquisition window of 30 to 50 milliseconds is helpful in obtaining sharp coronary MR angiograms.

Magnetic Field Strength and Imaging Sequence

Steady-state free-precession (SSFP) sequences are generally preferred to gradient-echo sequences at 1.5 T because the high T2/T1 ratio of the blood acts as an intrinsic contrast medium for SSFP coronary imaging, and helps to increase the blood signal on non–contrast-enhanced coronary MR angiography.[17,18] Higher magnetic field strength at 3 T is increasingly used for cardiac MR imaging, because high-field MR imaging can provide improved SNR.[19,20] The difficulties of 3-T cardiac MR imaging include increased off-resonance effect caused by magnetic field inhomogeneity and high specific adsorption rate. Because SSFP sequencing is susceptible to inhomogeneity of magnetic field and requires higher flip angles to obtain enough contrast between the blood and the myocardium, coronary MR angiography using SSFP acquisition is particularly challenging at higher field strength. Consequently, at 3 T gradient-echo sequences are generally preferred to SSFP for coronary MR angiography acquisition (**Fig. 5**).[21]

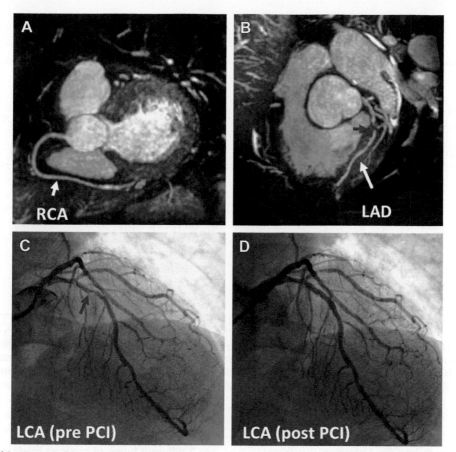

Fig. 4. In this 60-year-old man with chest pain on effort, coronary MR angiography (*A, B*) clearly demonstrated significant stenosis in the proximal LAD (*red arrow*). Invasive x-ray coronary angiography (*C*) confirmed significant stenosis in the proximal LAD (*red arrow*), which was successfully treated by percutaneous coronary intervention (PCI) (*D*). LCA, left coronary artery; RCA, right coronary artery.

Table 1
Comparison between systolic and diastolic coronary MR angiography acquisition

Diastolic Resting Period	Systolic Resting Period
Advantages	
Longer acquisition window (up to 100 ms) and potentially shorter imaging time in subjects with low and stable heart rate[a]	Less susceptible to heart rate variation during acquisition
Not susceptible to myocardial bridging	Adequate image quality in subjects with moderate to high heart rate
Disadvantages	
Image degradation when heart rate changes during acquisition	Shorter acquisition window (<50 ms) and relatively long acquisition time
No adequate rest period in patients with moderate to high heart rate	Susceptible to myocardial bridging

[a] A long acquisition window often results in substantial blurring of the coronary artery. Use a narrow acquisition window as much as possible to improve image quality of coronary MR angiography, by using multichannel coils for a high parallel imaging factor and abdominal belt for higher navigator efficiency.

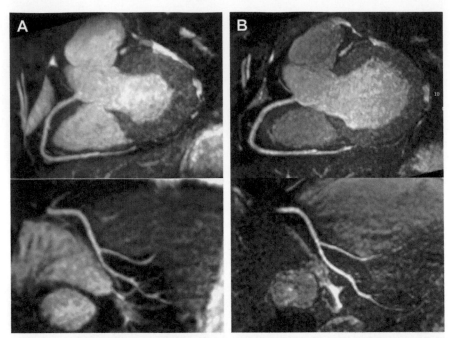

Fig. 5. Noncontrast free-breathing whole-heart coronary MR angiography acquired with a steady-state free-precession sequence at 1.5 T (*A*) and gradient-echo sequence at 3.0 T (*B*) in the same subject with normal coronary artery. For both magnetic field strengths, 32-channel coils, T2 preparation, and spectral fat-saturation inversion recovery (SPIR) were used. The image quality was comparable between these 2 coronary MR angiography images.

Preparation Pulses for Ensuring Sufficient Image Contrast

In contrast to 3D time-of-flight MR angiography of the cerebral arteries, the in-flow effect of the arterial blood is less prominent on coronary MR angiography. Therefore, suppression of the signal from the surrounding structures such as pericardial fat and myocardium is important to obtain sufficient arterial contrast on coronary MR angiography.[22,23] Spin preparations for coronary MR angiography usually include fat suppression and T2 preparation. Because the coronary artery is surrounded by epicardial fat, fat-saturation techniques such as short-tau inversion recovery (STIR) or spectral fat-saturation inversion recovery (SPIR) are essential to obtain diagnostic coronary MR angiography.[7] A T2-weighted magnetization preparation pulse is used to suppress myocardial signal.[24] T2 preparation is also useful for the suppression of venous blood signal in the epicardial veins.

Contrast Medium

The administration of gadolinium contrast medium helps to improve blood contrast and SNR on gradient-echo coronary MR angiography. There

are 3 different types of contrast medium currently available:

1. Extracellular contrast agent[25]
2. Intravascular contrast agent[26]
3. Slightly albumin-binding contrast agent[27]

Slightly albumin-binding agent exhibits relatively prolonged retention time in the blood and high relaxivities[28] while maintaining late enhancement abilities.[29]

When sufficient shortening of T1 relaxation time of the blood is achieved by administration of intravascular agent or high-dose slightly albumin-binding agent, gradient-echo MR angiography with inversion recovery prepulse exhibits high blood contrast and good fat saturation. In a recent single-center study by Yang and colleagues,[27] 3-T MR angiography data were acquired during a slow infusion of double-dose slightly albumin-binding contrast medium with inversion-recovery prepulse. The sensitivity and specificity of 3-T contrast-enhanced whole-heart coronary MR angiography was 94% and 82%, respectively, on a patient-based analysis, indicating that the diagnostic performance of 3-T contrast-enhanced whole-heart coronary MR angiography approaches that of 64-slice MDCT.

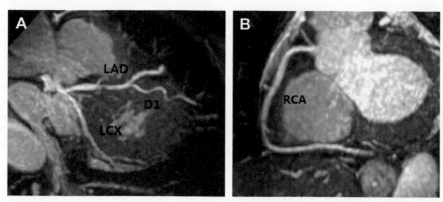

Fig. 6. Thin-slab maximum-intensity projection images of whole-heart coronary MR angiography acquired with a gradient-echo sequence in a subject with normal coronary artery at 3-T MR system for the left anterior descending artery (LAD) (*A*) and right coronary artery (RCA). (*B*) It should be noted that substantially good image quality is obtained even in the noncontrast 3-T whole-heart coronary MR angiography using T1-weighted gradient-echo sequence with T2 preparation and SPIR. D1, first diagonal branch; LCX, left circumflex artery.

Non–contrast-enhanced 3-T gradient-echo whole-heart coronary MR angiography can be acquired by using T2 preparation and SPIR fat saturation, with image quality comparable with that of 1.5-T SSFP acquisition. Although blood enhancement by extracellular contrast agent is smaller than that achieved by intravascular contrast agent because of the rapid extravasation to the interstitial space, acquisition of 3-T gradient-echo whole-heart coronary MR angiography after late gadolinium-enhancement MR imaging helps to increase the blood contrast (**Fig. 6**).

FUTURE PERSPECTIVE

Several limitations remain for coronary MR angiography in comparison with CT angiography, such as long scan times and limited spatial resolution and SNR. Respiratory navigator uses a simple linear motion model with a fixed correction factor of 0.6 to estimate and correct for respiratory-induced motion of the heart.[30] However, this simple model cannot compensate completely the bulk respiratory heart motion. Recently, direct respiratory motion estimation techniques of the heart with improved motion compensation performance were developed for free-breathing coronary MR angiography by using self-navigation and image-based navigation.[31,32] These techniques allow for coronary MR angiography data acquisition throughout most or all of the respiratory cycle, thereby significantly reducing scan time. Compressed sensing is a new image reconstruction method for accelerated acquisitions with incoherently undersampled k-space data.[33] Akçakaya and colleagues[34] used a B1-weighted compressed sensing technique for highly accelerated

submillimeter whole-heart coronary MR angiography. The image quality and SNR of the compressed sensing images were significantly higher than those of parallel imaging.[34] The implementation of compressed sensing and more sophisticated respiratory motion compensation techniques of the heart in clinical MR scanners may substantially improve the scan efficiency and spatial resolution of coronary MR angiography.

SUMMARY

Coronary MR angiography allows for noninvasive imaging of the coronary arteries without radiation exposure. Free-breathing whole-heart coronary MR angiography with navigator echo respiratory motion compensation, by using either 1.5-T SSFP or 3-T gradient-echo sequences, is the most widely used method for MR imaging of the coronary arteries. Spin preparations such as T2 preparation and fat saturation are essential to obtain sufficient blood contrast on coronary MR angiography. Further improvement of the blood contrast can be achieved by application of contrast medium. The abdominal belt and subject-specific narrow acquisition window are important in reducing motion blurring caused by respiration and cardiac contraction. Use of a high parallel imaging factor with 32-channel coils is highly beneficial in reducing the overall scan time and narrowing the acquisition window during the cardiac cycle. Further technical developments may allow acquisition of submillimeter whole-heart coronary MR angiography in a reduced scan time.

REFERENCES

1. Go AS, Mozaffarian D, Roger VL, et al. Executive summary: heart disease and stroke statistics-2014 update: a report from the American Heart Association. Circulation 2014;129:399–410.
2. Dewey M. Coronary CT versus MR angiography: pro CT-the role of CT angiography. Radiology 2011;258: 329–39.
3. Kato S, Kitagawa K, Ishida N, et al. Assessment of coronary artery disease using magnetic resonance coronary angiography: a national multicenter trial. J Am Coll Cardiol 2010;56:983–91.
4. Sakuma H, Ichikawa Y, Suzawa N, et al. Assessment of coronary arteries with total study time of less than 30 minutes by using whole-heart coronary MR angiography. Radiology 2005;237:316–21.
5. Jahnke C, Paetsch I, Nehrke K, et al. Rapid and complete coronary arterial tree visualization with magnetic resonance imaging: feasibility and diagnostic performance. Eur Heart J 2005;26:2313–9.
6. Sakuma H, Ichikawa Y, Chino S, et al. Detection of coronary artery stenosis with whole-heart coronary magnetic resonance angiography. J Am Coll Cardiol 2006;48:1946–50.
7. Nagata M, Kato S, Kitagawa K, et al. Diagnostic accuracy of 1.5-T unenhanced whole-heart coronary MR angiography performed with 32-channel cardiac coils: initial single-center experience. Radiology 2011;259:384–92.
8. Klein C, Gebker R, Kokocinski T, et al. Combined magnetic resonance coronary artery imaging, myocardial perfusion and late gadolinium enhancement in patients with suspected coronary artery disease. J Cardiovasc Magn Reson 2008;10:45.
9. Heer T, Reiter S, Höfling B, et al. Diagnostic performance of non-contrast-enhanced whole-heart magnetic resonance coronary angiography in combination with adenosine stress perfusion cardiac magnetic resonance imaging. Am Heart J 2013;166:999–1009.
10. McConnell MV, Khasgiwala VC, Savord BJ, et al. Comparison of respiratory suppression methods and navigator locations for MR coronary angiography. Am J Roentgenol 1997;168:1369–75.
11. Li D, Kaushikkar S, Haacke EM, et al. Coronary arteries: three-dimensional MR imaging with retrospective respiratory gating. Radiology 1996;201: 857–63.
12. Post JC, van Rossum AC, Hofman MB, et al. Three-dimensional respiratory-gated MR angiography of coronary arteries: comparison with conventional coronary angiography. Am J Roentgenol 1996;166: 1399–404.
13. Woodard PK, Li D, Haacke EM, et al. Detection of coronary stenoses on source and projection images using three-dimensional MR angiography with retrospective respiratory gating: preliminary experience. Am J Roentgenol 1998;170:883–8.
14. Ishida M, Schuster A, Takase S, et al. Impact of an abdominal belt on breathing patterns and scan efficiency in whole-heart coronary magnetic resonance angiography: comparison between the UK and Japan. J Cardiovasc Magn Reson 2011;13:71.
15. Kim WY, Stuber M, Kissinger KV, et al. Impact of bulk cardiac motion on right coronary MR angiography and vessel wall imaging. J Magn Reson Imaging 2001;14:383–90.
16. Plein S, Jones TR, Ridgway JP, et al. Three-dimensional coronary MR angiography performed with subject-specific cardiac acquisition windows and motion-adapted respiratory gating. Am J Roentgenol 2003;180:505–12.
17. Carr JC, Simonetti O, Bundy J, et al. Cine MR angiography of the heart with segmented true fast imaging with steady-state precession. Radiology 2001; 219:828–34.
18. McCarthy RM, Shea SM, Deshpande VS, et al. Coronary MR angiography: true FISP imaging improved by prolonging breath holds with preoxygenation in healthy volunteers. Radiology 2003;227:283–8.
19. Stuber M, Botnar RM, Fischer SE, et al. Preliminary report on in vivo coronary MRA at 3 Tesla in humans. Magn Reson Med 2002;48:425–9.
20. Sommer T, Hackenbroch M, Hofer U, et al. Coronary MR angiography at 3.0 T versus that at 1.5 T: initial results in patients suspected of having coronary artery disease. Radiology 2005;234:718–25.
21. Kaul MG, Stork A, Bansmann PM, et al. Evaluation of balanced steady-state free precession (TrueFISP) and K-space segmented gradient echo sequences for 3D coronary MR angiography with navigator gating at 3 Tesla. Rofo 2004;176:1560–5.
22. Manning WJ, Li W, Edelman RR. A preliminary report comparing magnetic resonance coronary angiography with conventional angiography. N Engl J Med 1993;328:828–32.
23. Li D, Paschal CB, Haacke EM, et al. Coronary arteries: three-dimensional MR imaging with fat saturation and magnetization transfer contrast. Radiology 1993;187:401–6.
24. Botnar RM, Stuber M, Danias PG, et al. Improved coronary artery definition with T2-weighted, free-breathing, three-dimensional coronary MRA. Circulation 1999;99:3139–48.
25. Regenfus M, Ropers D, Achenbach S, et al. Noninvasive detection of coronary artery stenosis using contrast-enhanced three-dimensional breath-hold magnetic resonance coronary angiography. J Am Coll Cardiol 2000;36:44–50.
26. Tang L, Merkle N, Schär M, et al. Volume-targeted and whole-heart coronary magnetic resonance angiography using an intravascular contrast agent. J Magn Reson Imaging 2009;30:1191–6.

27. Yang Q, Li K, Liu X, et al. Contrast-enhanced whole-heart coronary magnetic resonance angiography at 3.0-T: a comparative study with X-ray angiography in a single center. J Am Coll Cardiol 2009;54:69–76.

28. Laurent S, Elst LV, Muller RN. Comparative study of the physicochemical properties of six clinical low molecular weight gadolinium contrast agents. Contrast Media Mol Imaging 2006;1:128–37.

29. Krombach GA, Hahnen C, Lodemann KP, et al. Gd-BOPTA for assessment of myocardial viability on MRI: changes of T1 value and their impact on delayed enhancement. Eur Radiol 2009;19: 2136–46.

30. Stuber M, Botnar RM, Danias PG, et al. Submillimeter three-dimensional coronary MR angiography with real-time navigator correction: comparison of navigator locations. Radiology 1999;212:579–87.

31. Piccini D, Littmann A, Nielles-Vallespin S, et al. Respiratory self-navigation for whole-heart bright-blood coronary MRI: methods for robust isolation and automatic segmentation of the blood pool. Magn Reson Med 2012;68:571–9.

32. Henningsson M, Koken P, Stehning C, et al. Whole-heart coronary MR angiography with 2D self-navigated image reconstruction. Magn Reson Med 2012;67:437–45.

33. Akçakaya M, Rayatzadeh H, Basha TA, et al. Accelerated late gadolinium enhancement cardiac MR imaging with isotropic spatial resolution using compressed sensing: initial experience. Radiology 2012;264:691–9.

34. Akçakaya M, Basha TA, Chan RH, et al. Accelerated isotropic sub-millimeter whole-heart coronary MRI: compressed sensing versus parallel imaging. Magn Reson Med 2014;71:815–22.

Rings and Slings Revisited

Brandon M. Smith, MD[a],*, Jimmy C. Lu, MD[a,b], Adam L. Dorfman, MD[a,b],
Maryam Ghadimi Mahani, MD[b,c], Prachi P. Agarwal, MBBS, MS[c]

KEYWORDS

• MR imaging • Vascular ring • Pulmonary sling • Pediatrics

KEY POINTS

- Vascular rings and pulmonary artery slings present with symptoms of tracheal and esophageal compression during infancy and childhood.
- Double aortic arch and right aortic arch with aberrant left subclavian artery and left patent ductus arteriosus (PDA) are the 2 most common types of vascular ring.
- Atretic segments cannot be directly visualized on MR imaging, but their presence can be inferred from other indirect imaging signs.
- MR imaging/magnetic resonance angiography (MRA) can diagnose these vascular anomalies and evaluate the airway and esophagus without the use of ionizing radiation.

INTRODUCTION

Vascular rings and pulmonary artery slings are rare congenital anomalies of the aortic arch branches or pulmonary arteries that often present with symptoms of tracheal or esophageal compression during childhood. Diagnosis of these conditions can be made using various imaging modalities, including radiography, esophagography, echocardiography, CT, and MR imaging.[1] The purpose of this review is to highlight the advantages of MR imaging for the diagnosis of vascular rings and pulmonary artery slings and to provide an insight into the diagnosis of specific vascular ring types using case examples.

ADVANTAGES OF MR IMAGING

MR imaging possesses unique advantages over other imaging modalities in the diagnosis of vascular rings and pulmonary artery slings. Chest radiography can detect a right aortic arch or tracheal compression, and barium esophagography may demonstrate esophageal compression,[2] but these modalities do not directly image vascular structures and cannot provide conclusive anatomic diagnosis, which can be essential for surgical planning.[3] Echocardiography can diagnose aortic arch sidedness and branching pattern, double aortic arches, and pulmonary artery anatomy. Tracheal and esophageal compression cannot be evaluated, however, and due to suboptimal acoustic windows may limit diagnostic accuracy for vascular rings.[4] Angiography can image patent vascular structures but cannot demonstrate tracheal and esophageal compression, requires invasive vascular access with a potential for complications, and requires ionizing radiation and nephrotoxic contrast agent.

Disclosures: No financial relationships or conflicts of interest to disclose.

[a] Division of Pediatric Cardiology, Department of Pediatrics and Communicable Diseases, University of Michigan, 1540 East Hospital Drive, Ann Arbor, MI 48109, USA; [b] Division of Pediatric Radiology, Department of Radiology, University of Michigan, 1500 East Medical Center Drive, Ann Arbor, MI 48109, USA; [c] Division of Cardiothoracic Radiology, Department of Radiology, University of Michigan, 1500 East Medical Center Drive, Ann Arbor, MI 48109, USA
* Corresponding author. University of Michigan Congenital Heart Center, C.S. Mott Children's Hospital, 1540 East Hospital Drive, Ann Arbor, MI 48109-4204.
E-mail address: bsmi@med.umich.edu

Magn Reson Imaging Clin N Am 23 (2015) 127–135
http://dx.doi.org/10.1016/j.mric.2014.09.011
1064-9689/15/$ – see front matter © 2015 Elsevier Inc. All rights reserved.

Due to the ability to delineate vascular anatomy with multiplanar and 3-D reconstruction, and simultaneously demonstrate tracheal and esophageal compression, CT and MR imaging have become the preferred imaging modalities for the diagnosis of vascular rings and pulmonary artery slings. MRA can demonstrate vascular anatomy similar to CT without using ionizing radiation, which is particularly desirable in this young population.[5]

MR IMAGING PROTOCOL

MR imaging protocol for vascular ring and pulmonary artery sling evaluation typically consists of gadolinium-enhanced angiography and ECG-gated black blood and bright blood sequences.

- Black blood imaging in axial and oblique coronal (oriented along the trachea) planes is useful for assessment of vascular anatomy, tracheobronchial tree, and esophagus.
- Unless contraindicated, 3-D gadolinium-enhanced MRA provides comprehensive assessment of vascular anatomy.
- ECG and respiratory navigator-gated 3-D steady-state free precession (SSFP) imaging can simultaneously assess vascular, airway, and esophageal anatomy in a 3-D data set without the need for gadolinium.

VASCULAR RINGS

A vascular ring is defined as an abnormality of the aortic arch, its branches, or remnants that results in encircling of the trachea and esophagus with variable degrees of compression. Vascular rings represent 1% to 3% of congenital cardiac anomalies[6] and may remain asymptomatic or present at various times throughout childhood with stridor, dyspnea, chronic cough, wheezing, recurrent respiratory infection, or dysphagia, which may be relieved by surgery.[7]

Normal Aortic Arch Development

Normal aortic arch development involves variable regression of 6 paired aortic arches from the aortic sac to the paired dorsal aortae. The first, second, and third arches form parts of the maxillary, stapedial, and common carotid arteries, respectively.[8] Remnants of the fourth arch form the distal left aortic arch and proximal right subclavian artery. The fifth arches usually regress, and the sixth arches form parts of the pulmonary arteries and distal ductus arteriosus. The spectrum of aortic arch anomalies and vascular rings can be easily understood using the Edwards hypothetical double arch system (**Fig. 1**). Normal left arch anatomy

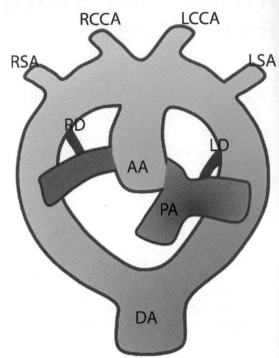

Fig. 1. Schematic diagram of Edward's hypothetical double aortic arch. The 2 arches give rise to the respective carotid and subclavian arteries and ductus arteriosus. AA, ascending aorta; DA, descending aorta; LCCA, left common carotid artery; LD, left ductus arteriosus; LSA, left subclavian artery; PA, pulmonary artery; RCCA, right common carotid artery; RD, right ductus arteriosus; RSA, right subclavian artery.

occurs after involution of the distal right fourth arch and regression of the right ductus (**Fig. 2**). Abnormal patterns of regression of these paired aortic arches can result in a vascular ring.

Aortic arch sidedness is defined by the location of the aortic arch in relation to the trachea (left, right, or double) as it passes over the mainstem bronchus (**Fig. 3**).[9] On echocardiography and angiography, this determination is indirect and may be inaccurate. MR imaging directly visualizes both the aorta and tracheobronchial tree, thus allowing conclusive diagnosis.

The spectrum of vascular rings (**Table 1**), with their distinctive MR imaging appearance, is described later.

Double Aortic Arch

Double aortic arch, a persistence of the right and left 4th embryonic arches, is the most common form of vascular ring, comprising approximately 50% of cases, and often presents from birth through childhood with respiratory symptoms,

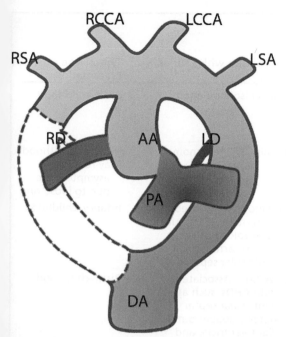

Fig. 2. Schematic diagram of development of the left aortic arch with normal brachiocephalic branching. The right arch (between the right subclavian artery and descending aorta) involutes along with regression of the right ductus arteriosus (*dashed lines*). AA, ascending aorta; DA, descending aorta; LCCA, left common carotid artery; LD, left ductus arteriosus; LSA, left subclavian artery; PA, pulmonary artery; RCCA, right common carotid artery; RD, right ductus arteriosus; RSA, right subclavian artery.

such as stridor, asthma, and recurrent croup.[8] Association with other cardiac anomalies is uncommon, but approximately 10% to 15% of patients may have a chromosome 22q11 deletion.[10]

When both arches are patent (whether codominant or asymmetric in size), imaging diagnosis is straightforward (**Fig. 4**), and associated tracheal compression is often present. Dominant right arch with hypoplastic or atretic left arch is most common (prevalence 70%–75%[1]), whereas dominant left arch or codominant aortic arches are less common (prevalence 20% and 5%, respectively[11]). Determining the dominant aortic arch is important for surgical planning, because thoracotomy is performed on the side of the nondominant arch.[12] Also, it is important to recognize a hypoplastic but patent arch, because a thoracoscopic approach may not be preferred with a patent nondominant arch due to risk of bleeding.

The imaging diagnosis of double aortic arch with distal left arch atresia can be more challenging. The embryologic basis for this anomaly is atresia (with a residual fibrous cord) between the left subclavian artery and descending aorta. If the atresia occurs between the left ductus and left subclavian artery, both the atretic cord and ligamentum attach to the descending aortic diverticulum (**Fig. 5**) and need to be addressed at surgery. If the regression abnormality is in the segment after the ductus, however, only the fibrous cord completes the ring and attaches to the aortic diverticulum. The ductus then arises from the anterior left arch (**Fig. 6**).

Right aortic arch with mirror image branching also involves regression of the segment after the ductus (**Fig. 7**), with the ductus arising from the innominate artery. The only difference from the previously described double aortic arch is that the involution is complete, with no residual fibrous cord and thus no vascular ring. On imaging, a double aortic arch with atretic left arch can mimic a right aortic arch with mirror image branching because the atretic segment itself cannot be directly visualized. The 2 most important differentiating features seen in a double aortic arch include the 4-vessel sign (symmetric arrangement of the carotids and subclavian arteries from the 2 arches) and a diverticulum from the descending aorta.[13]

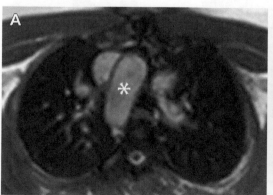
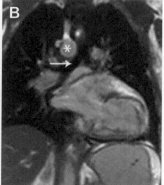

Fig. 3. Axial (*A*) and coronal (*B*) cine SSFP MR images demonstrate a right aortic arch (*asterisk*) crossing over the right main stem bronchus (*arrow*).

Table 1
Vascular ring and pulmonary artery sling types

Vascular Ring Type	Total Vascular Rings (%)	Association with CHD or Syndromes	Typical Age at Presentation
DAA[1,8]	50	Usually isolated anomaly	Birth–childhood
Right dominant	70–75 of DAA		
Left dominant	20 of DAA		
Codominant	5 of DAA		
Right aortic arch with aberrant left subclavian[4,14,15]	30	Usually isolated anomaly	Infancy–adulthood May remain asymptomatic due to loose ring
Right aortic arch with mirror image branching and retroesophageal ductus arteriosus[19]	5	Commonly associated with other CHDs, such as tetralogy of Fallot, truncus arteriosus, ventricular septal defect	Infancy–childhood
Circumflex aortic arch[20,21]	Rare	50%–60% Associated with CHDs, such as ventricular septal defect, double-outlet right ventricle, and coarctation	Birth–childhood

Abbreviations: CHD, congenital heart disease; DAA, double aortic arch.

Another subjective sign is a more posteriorly positioned incomplete left arch compared with the innominate artery in a right arch with mirror image branching (**Fig. 8**). Similarly, a double aortic arch with atresia between the left carotid and left subclavian arteries can simulate the imaging appearance of right arch with retro esophageal diverticulum of Kommerell.

Right Aortic Arch with Aberrant Left Subclavian Artery and Left Ductus Arteriosus

Right aortic arch with aberrant left subclavian artery and left ductus arteriosus is the second most common form of vascular ring, comprising approximately 30% of cases,[4] and is also usually an isolated finding, with a 5% to 15% prevalence of associated congenital heart disease.[14] The

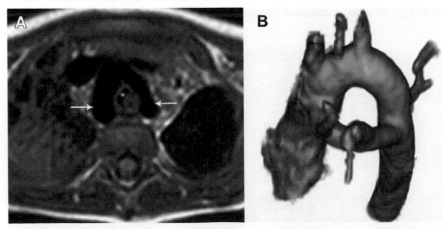

Fig. 4. Double aortic arch. Axial black blood image (*A*) demonstrates bilateral patent aortic arches (*arrows*), with the right arch the larger of the 2. Note the narrowed trachea (*asterisk*). The complete ring formed by the 2 patent arches is well seen on the volume-rendered reconstruction from the gadolinium-enhanced MRA (*B*).

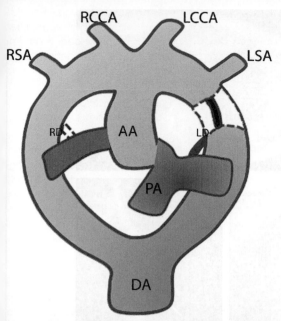

Fig. 5. Schematic diagram showing embryologic basis of a double aortic arch with distal left arch atresia. Due to abnormal regression between the left ductus and left subclavian artery, both the atretic cord and ductus attach to the descending aortic diverticulum. AA, ascending aorta; DA, descending aorta; LCCA, left common carotid artery; LD, left ductus arteriosus; LSA, left subclavian artery; PA, pulmonary artery; RCCA, right common carotid artery; RD, right ductus arteriosus; RSA, right subclavian artery.

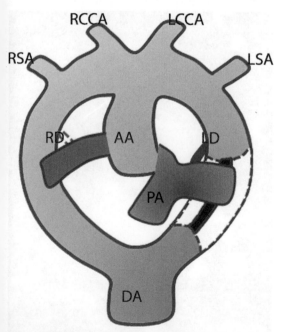

Fig. 6. Schematic diagram showing embryologic basis of a double aortic arch with distal left arch atresia. Due to atresia of the segment after the ductus, only the fibrous cord completes the ring and attaches to the aortic diverticulum. AA, ascending aorta; DA, descending aorta; LCCA, left common carotid artery; LD, left ductus arteriosus; LSA, left subclavian artery; PA, pulmonary artery; RCCA, right common carotid artery; RD, right ductus arteriosus; RSA, right subclavian artery.

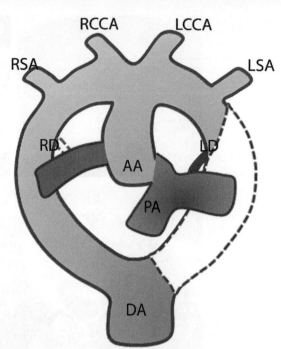

Fig. 7. Schematic diagram showing embryologic basis of a right aortic arch with mirror image branching. There is complete involution of the segment (*dashed lines*) after the ductus with the ductus arising from the innominate artery. AA, ascending aorta; DA, descending aorta; LCCA, left common carotid artery; LD, left ductus arteriosus; LSA, left subclavian artery; PA, pulmonary artery; RCCA, right common carotid artery; RD, right ductus arteriosus; RSA, right subclavian artery.

presentation is variable, with approximately 40% of patients experiencing symptoms.[15] Right aortic arch with aberrant left subclavian artery results from regression of the left aortic arch segment between the left common carotid and subclavian arteries (**Fig. 9**). Although the ligamentum arteriosum cannot be directly identified, its position can be inferred by noting an increased caliber of the proximal left subclavian artery from the descending aorta (referred to as Kommerell diverticulum) (**Fig. 10**). Kommerell diverticulum is related to flow from the PDA through the proximal aberrant left subclavian artery during fetal circulation. This increased flow creates the caliber difference of the proximal aberrant left subclavian artery with tapering to a normal caliber[9] distal to the presumed site of ductus arteriosus. In the absence of a left ductus, the aberrant left subclavian artery has uniform caliber throughout (**Fig. 11**) and is often seen in association with conotruncal anomalies. In these circumstances, there is no vascular ring.

If symptomatic, usually presenting from childhood to adult age with swallowing difficulty rather

132

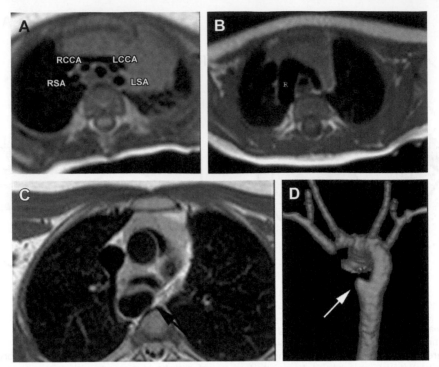

Fig. 8. Double aortic arch and distal left arch atresia. Axial black blood images (*A–C*) and volume-rendered reconstruction from gadolinium-enhanced MRA (*D*) depict the anatomy of the vascular ring. Note the 4-vessel sign with symmetric arrangement of carotid and subclavian arteries from the ipsilateral arches (*A*). Slightly more caudally (*B*), a dominant right (R) arch is seen with atresia of distal left arch. The atretic arch itself is not directly visualized. Also, note the diverticulum (*arrow*) from the aorta (*C, D*). LCCA, left common carotid artery; LSA, left subclavian artery; RCCA, right common carotid artery; RSA, right subclavian artery.

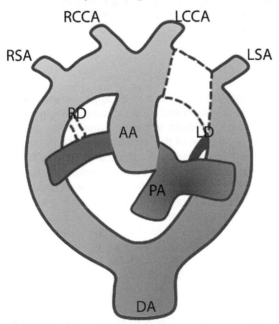

Fig. 9. Schematic diagram showing embryologic basis of a right aortic arch with retroesophageal diverticulum of Kommerell. There is involution of the segment (*dashed lines*) of left arch between the left carotid and left subclavian artery with regression of the right ductus. AA, ascending aorta; DA, descending aorta; LCCA, left common carotid artery; LD, left ductus arteriosus; LSA, left subclavian artery; PA, pulmonary artery; RCCA, right common carotid artery; RD, right ductus arteriosus; RSA, right subclavian artery.

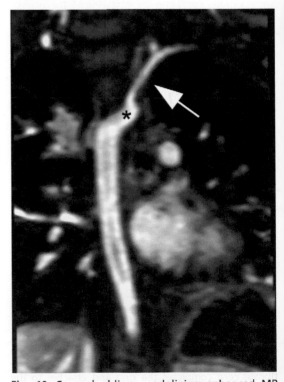

Fig. 10. Coronal oblique gadolinium-enhanced MR angiogram of a right aortic arch with retroesophageal diverticulum of Kommerell (*asterisk*). Note the change in caliber of the aberrant left subclavian artery (*arrow*) after the diverticulum (*asterisk*) at the presumed site of left ductus. This anomaly comprises a vascular ring.

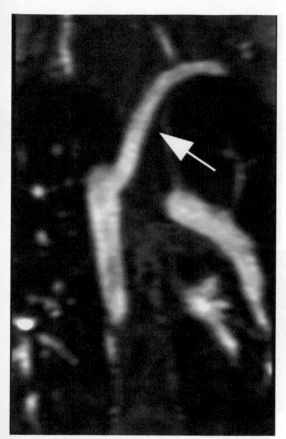

Fig. 11. Coronal oblique gadolinium-enhanced MR angiogram of a right aortic arch with aberrant left subclavian artery and no left ductus. Note the uniform caliber of the left subclavian artery (*arrow*) and the absence of retroesophageal diverticulum of Kommerell. This entity does not constitute a vascular ring.

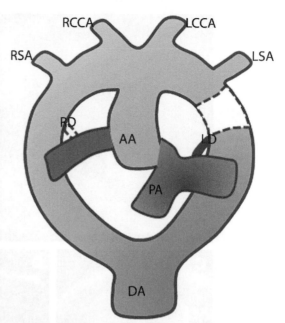

Fig. 12. Schematic diagram showing embryologic basis of a right aortic arch with mirror image branching and retroesophageal ductus. There is involution of the segment (*dashed lines*) of left arch between the left ductus and left subclavian artery. AA, ascending aorta; DA, descending aorta; LCCA, left common carotid artery; LD, left ductus arteriosus; LSA, left subclavian artery; PA, pulmonary artery; RCCA, right common carotid artery; RD, right ductus arteriosus; RSA, right subclavian artery.

than respiratory distress, surgical division of the ligamentum arteriosum via thoracotomy is the usual management.[3,7] Rarely, a left aortic arch with aberrant right subclavian artery and right-sided ductus arteriosus or ligamentum arteriosum may cause a mirror image vascular ring of the right aortic arch with aberrant left subclavian artery.[16]

Right Aortic Arch with Mirror Image Branching and Retroesophageal Patent Ductus Arteriosus

Right aortic arch with mirror image branching has a reported 66% to 98% reported incidence of associated congenital heart disease accompanying intracardiac abnormalities, such as tetralogy of Fallot and truncus arteriosus.[2,17,18] This classically does not form a vascular ring (see **Fig. 7**). Infrequently, however, a right aortic arch with mirror image branching may form a vascular ring

due to a ductus or ligamentum arteriosum from the proximal descending aorta that courses posterior to the trachea and esophagus prior to inserting into the left pulmonary artery (**Fig. 12**).[19] MR imaging and MRA again aid in identification of an aortic dimple (tapered blind-ending outpouching), which, in conjunction with symptoms or evidence of tracheal or esophageal compression, help confirm the diagnosis. Division of the ductus/ligamentum arteriosum is the treatment of this lesion.[16] Because this lesion is less common than double aortic arch with atretic left arch, however, surgeons should also inspect for an atretic left aortic arch segment, which, if present, also needs to be divided to relieve the ring.

Circumflex Aortic Arch

Circumflex aortic arch is a rare vascular anomaly consisting of an aortic arch with a retroesophageal segment and proximal descending aorta contralateral to the arch (**Fig. 13**). A vascular ring occurs with a right circumflex aortic arch and left PDA from the descending aorta to the left pulmonary artery or with a left circumflex aortic arch and right

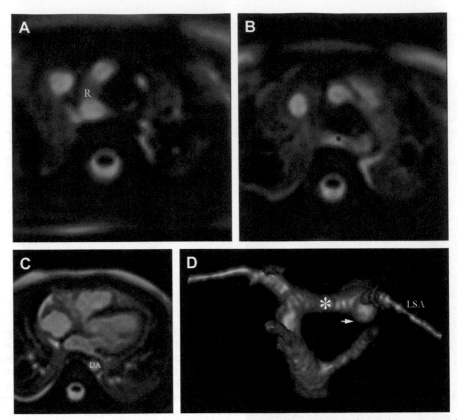

Fig. 13. Circumflex right aortic arch with left descending aorta and aberrant left subclavian artery (LSA). Axial cine SSFP images (*A–C*) demonstrate circumflex right arch (R) with retroesophageal (*asterisk*) segment and left descending aorta (DA). The left subclavian artery is aberrant and arises as the last branch. The retroesophageal vessel is the arch itself, however, and not the subclavian artery with a diverticulum of Kommerell. Volume-rendered image (*D*) demonstrates the anatomy of the circumflex right arch with retroesophageal (*asterisk*) segment and the aberrant left subclavian artery (LSA) with a diverticulum of Kommerell (*arrow*).

PDA. An aberrant subclavian artery may also occur, although this entity differs from a right arch and aberrant left subclavian artery with diverticulum of Kommerell in that the aorta itself is retroesophageal and not the subclavian artery. There is 50% to 60% prevalence for additional cardiac anomalies.[20,21] Chest radiography and echocardiography have shown poor sensitivity for this diagnosis, whereas MR imaging can accurately define the aortic arch anatomy for surgical planning.[20]

PULMONARY ARTERY SLINGS

A pulmonary artery sling is an anomalous origin of the left pulmonary artery from the right pulmonary artery with a course between the trachea and esophagus (**Fig. 14**). Presenting symptoms, often during the neonatal period or infancy, include stridor, respiratory distress, and recurrent respiratory infection.[22] A type I sling is just above the carina at T4-5 level and is usually associated with a normal

trachea. Type II slings are located more caudally adjacent to a low T-shaped carina at T5-6 level and often have long segment tracheal stenosis due to complete cartilaginous tracheal rings,[22,23] resulting in an O-shaped trachea with absent

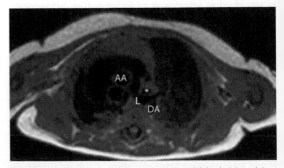

Fig. 14. Pulmonary artery sling. Axial black blood image demonstrates left pulmonary artery (L) arising from the proximal right pulmonary artery and coursing posterior to the trachea (*asterisk*). AA, ascending aorta, DA, descending aorta.

pars membranacea. Because the tracheal obstruction is primary and not just by extrinsic compression, the surgical treatment involves tracheoplasty in addition to addressing the vascular abnormality. MR imaging can clearly demonstrate the origin and course of the anomalous left pulmonary artery.[24] Although airways can be visualized on MR imaging, CT may be better suited for precise airway assessment.

SUMMARY

Vascular rings and pulmonary artery slings are a rare group of vascular anomalies, often presenting with symptoms of tracheal or esophageal compression during childhood. Despite the number of variations, these anomalies can be better appreciated with an understanding of their embryology and can be comprehensively evaluated with MR imaging, without ionizing radiation.

REFERENCES

1. Dillman JR, Attili AK, Agarwal PP, et al. Common and uncommon vascular rings and slings: a multimodality review. Pediatr Radiol 2011;41(11):1440–54 [quiz: 1489–90].
2. Hernanz-Schulman M. Vascular rings: a practical approach to imaging diagnosis. Pediatr Radiol 2005;35(10):961–79.
3. van Son JA, Julsrud PR, Hagler DJ, et al. Surgical treatment of vascular rings: the Mayo Clinic experience. Mayo Clin Proc 1993;68(11):1056–63.
4. van Son JA, Julsrud PR, Hagler DJ, et al. Imaging strategies for vascular rings. Ann Thorac Surg 1994;57(3):604–10.
5. Azarow KS, Pearl RH, Hoffman MA, et al. Vascular ring: does magnetic resonance imaging replace angiography? Ann Thorac Surg 1992;53(5):882–5.
6. Marmon LM, Bye MR, Haas JM, et al. Vascular rings and slings: long-term follow-up of pulmonary function. J Pediatr Surg 1984;19(6):683–92.
7. Oddone M, Granata C, Vercellino N, et al. Multi-modality evaluation of the abnormalities of the aortic arches in children: techniques and imaging spectrum with emphasis on MRI. Pediatr Radiol 2005;35(10):947–60.
8. Kellenberger CJ. Aortic arch malformations. Pediatr Radiol 2010;40(6):876–84.
9. Weinberg PM. Aortic arch anomalies. J Cardiovasc Magn Reson 2006;8(4):633–43.
10. McElhinney DB, Clark BJ 3rd, Weinberg PM, et al. Association of chromosome 22q11 deletion with iso-

11. Kimura-Hayama ET, Melendez G, Mendizabal AL, et al. Uncommon congenital and acquired aortic diseases: role of multidetector CT angiography. Radiographics 2010;30(1):79–98.
12. McFaul R, Millard P, Nowicki E. Vascular rings necessitating right thoracotomy. J Thorac Cardiovasc Surg 1981;82(2):306–9.
13. Schlesinger AE, Krishnamurthy R, Sena LM, et al. Incomplete double aortic arch with atresia of the distal left arch: distinctive imaging appearance. AJR Am J Roentgenol 2005;184(5):1634–9.
14. Shuford WH, Sybers RG. The aortic arch and its malformations; with emphasis on the angiographic features. Springfield (IL): Thomas; 1973.
15. Suh YJ, Kim GB, Kwon BS, et al. Clinical course of vascular rings and risk factors associated with mortality. Korean Circ J 2012;42(4):252–8.
16. Kussman BD, Geva T, McGowan FX. Cardiovascular causes of airway compression. Paediatr Anaesth 2004;14(1):60–74.
17. Zidere V, Tsapakis EG, Huggon IC, et al. Right aortic arch in the fetus. Ultrasound Obstet Gynecol 2006;28(7):876–81.
18. Kersting-Sommerhoff BA, Sechtem UP, Fisher MR, et al. MR imaging of congenital anomalies of the aortic arch. AJR Am J Roentgenol 1987;149(1):9–13.
19. McElhinney DB, Hoydu AK, Gaynor JW, et al. Patterns of right aortic arch and mirror-image branching of the brachiocephalic vessels without associated anomalies. Pediatr Cardiol 2001;22(4):285–91.
20. Philip S, Chen SY, Wu MH, et al. Retroesophageal aortic arch: diagnostic and therapeutic implications of a rare vascular ring. Int J Cardiol 2001;79(2–3):133–41.
21. Ergin MA, Jayaram N, LaCorte M. Left aortic arch and right descending aorta: diagnostic and therapeutic implications of a rare type of vascular ring. Ann Thorac Surg 1981;31(1):82–5.
22. Pawade A, de Leval MR, Elliott MJ, et al. Pulmonary artery sling. Ann Thorac Surg 1992;54(5):967–70.
23. Berdon WE. Rings, slings, and other things: vascular compression of the infant trachea updated from the midcentury to the millennium–the legacy of Robert E. Gross, MD, and Edward B. D. Neuhauser, MD. Radiology 2000;216(3):624–32.
24. Eichhorn J, Fink C, Delorme S, et al. Rings, slings and other vascular abnormalities. Ultrafast computed tomography and magnetic resonance angiography in pediatric cardiology. Z Kardiol 2004;93(3):201–8.

pary membranosa. Because the tracheal
obstruction is primary and not just by extrinsic
compression, the surgical treatment involves tracheoplasty in addition to addressing the vascular
abnormality. MR imaging can clearly demonstrate
the origin and course of the anomalous left pulmonary artery. Although airways can be visualized
on MR imaging, CT may be better suited for precise airway assessment.

SUMMARY

Vascular rings and pulmonary artery slings are a
rare group of vascular anomalies, often more often
with symptoms of respiratory or, though due
compromise. A common cause of the number of vascular anomalies can be better
appreciated with anatomic delineation of the anatomy
ology and can be comprehensively displayed with
MR imaging, without ionizing radiation.

REFERENCES

Index

Note: Page numbers of article titles are in **boldface** type.

Magn Reson Imaging Clin N Am 23 (2015) 137–140
http://dx.doi.org/10.1016/S1064-9689(14)00127-5
1064-9689/15/$ – see front matter © 2015 Elsevier Inc. All rights reserved.

Moving?

Make sure your subscription moves with you!

To notify us of your new address, find your **Clinics Account Number** (located on your mailing label above your name), and contact customer service at:

Email: journalscustomerservice-usa@elsevier.com

800-654-2452 (subscribers in the U.S. & Canada)
314-447-8871 (subscribers outside of the U.S. & Canada)

Fax number: 314-447-8029

Elsevier Health Sciences Division
Subscription Customer Service
3251 Riverport Lane
Maryland Heights, MO 63043

*To ensure uninterrupted delivery of your subscription, please notify us at least 4 weeks in advance of move.

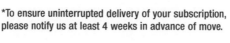

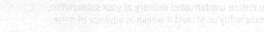

Printed and bound by CPI Group (UK) Ltd, Croydon, CR0 4YY

03/10/2024

01040374-0010